PRETEST®

Physiology

Notice

Medicine is an ever-changing science. As new research and clinical experience broaden our knowledge, changes in treatment and drug therapy are required. The editors and the publisher of this work have checked with sources believed to be reliable in their efforts to provide information that is complete and generally in accord with the standards accepted at the time of publication. However, in view of the possibility of human error or changes in medical sciences, neither the editors nor the publisher nor any other party who has been involved in the preparation or publication of this work warrants that the information contained herein is in every respect accurate or complete, and they are not responsible for any errors or omissions or for the results obtained from use of such information. Readers are encouraged to confirm the information contained herein with other sources. For example and in particular, readers are advised to check the product information sheet included in the package of each drug they plan to administer to be certain that the information contained in this book is accurate and that changes have not been made in the recommended dose or in the contraindications for administration. This recommendation is of particular importance in connection with new or infrequently used drugs.

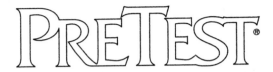

Physiology

PreTest®
Self-Assessment
and Review

Eighth Edition

Edited by
James P. Ryan, Ph.D.
Professor and Deputy Chair
Department of Physiology
Temple University School of Medicine
Philadelphia, Pennsylvania

Ronald F. Tuma, Ph.D.
Professor and Chair
Department of Physiology
Temple University School of Medicine
Philadelphia, Pennsylvania

 McGraw-Hill
Health Professions Division
PreTest® Series

New York   St. Louis   San Francisco   Auckland
Bogotá   Caracas   Lisbon   London   Madrid
Mexico City   Milan   Montreal   New Delhi
San Juan   Singapore   Sydney   Tokyo   Toronto

McGraw-Hill

A Division of The **McGraw·Hill** Companies

Physiology: PreTest® Self-Assessment and Review, Eighth Edition
Copyright © 1996, 1993, 1991, 1988, 1986, 1983, 1980, 1976 by the McGraw-Hill
Companies, Inc. All rights reserved. Printed in the United States of America. Except as
permitted under the Copyright Act of 1976, no part of this publication may be repro-
duced or distributed in any form or by any means, or stored in a data base or retrieval
system, without the prior written permission of the publisher.

1 2 3 4 5 6 7 8 9 0   DOCDOC   9 9 8 7 6 5

ISBN 0-07-052085-2

The editors were Gail Gavert and Bruce MacGregor.
The production supervisor was Gyl A. Favours.
This book was set in Times Roman by Digitype.
R.R. Donnelley & Sons was printer and binder.

Library of Congress Cataloging-in-Publication Data
Physiology : PreTest self-assessment and review. — 8th ed. / edited by James P.
Ryan, Ronald F. Tuma.
    p.   cm.
    Includes bibliographical references.
    ISBN 0-07-052085-2
    1. Human physiology—Examinations, questions, etc.   I. Ryan, James P.
    II. Tuma, Ronald F. (Ronald Franklin)
    [DNLM: 1. Physiology—examination questions.   QT 18.2 P578 1996]
  QP40.P47   1996
  612'.0076—dc20
DNLM/DLC
for Library of Congress   95–3618

Contents

Introduction

Each *PreTest® Self-Assessment and Review* allows medical students to comprehensively and conveniently assess and review their knowledge of a particular basic science, in this instance Physiology. The 500 questions parallel the format and degree of difficulty of the questions found in the United States Medical Licensing Examination (USMLE) Step 1. Practicing physicians who want to hone their skills before USMLE Step 3 or recertification may find this to be a good beginning in their review process.

Each question is accompanied by an answer, a paragraph explanation, and a specific page reference to an appropriate textbook or journal article. A bibliography listing sources can be found following the last chapter of this text.

An effective way to use this PreTest is to allow yourself one minute to answer each question in a given chapter. As you proceed, indicate your answer beside each question. By following this suggestion, you approximate the time limits imposed by the Step.

After you finish going through the questions in the section, spend as much time as you need verifying your answers and carefully reading the explanations provided. Pay special attention to the explanations for the questions you answered incorrectly—but read *every* explanation. The authors of this material have designed the explanations to reinforce and supplement the information tested by the questions. If you feel you need further information about the material covered, consult and study the references indicated.

PRETEST®

Physiology

Cellular Physiology

DIRECTIONS: Each question below contains five suggested responses. Select the **one best** response to each question.

1. Which of the following characteristics of an axon is most dependent on its diameter?

(A) Its resting potential
(B) The duration of its refractory period
(C) The conduction velocity of its action potential
(D) The overshoot of its action potential
(E) The activity of its sodium-potassium pump

2. A red blood cell will shrink by the greatest amount when it is placed in a solution containing

(A) 300 mM urea
(B) 200 mM NaCl
(C) 200 mM glucose
(D) 200 mM urea and 200 mMolar glucose
(E) 100 mM $CaCl_2$

3. If the extracellular K^+ concentration is increased from 4 meq/L to 10 meq/L,

(A) the membrane potential will become more negative
(B) the sodium conductance will increase
(C) the potassium conductance will increase
(D) the membrane will become more excitable
(E) the Na-K pump will become inactivated

4. Which one of the following is accomplished by secondary active transport?

(A) The secretion of H^+ by the renal distal tubule
(B) The sequestering of Ca^{2+} by the sarcoplasmic reticulum
(C) The reabsorption of HPO_4^{2-} by the renal proximal tubule
(D) The removal of Na^+ from a nerve axon
(E) The flow of K^+ out of a cardiac myocyte

5. Membrane excitability will be increased by the greatest amount by

(A) increasing extracellular Na^+
(B) increasing extracellular K^+
(C) decreasing extracellular Cl^-
(D) decreasing extracellular Ca^{2+}
(E) decreasing extracellular H^+

6. The resting potential of a nerve membrane is primarily dependent on the concentration gradient of

(A) potassium
(B) sodium
(C) calcium
(D) chloride
(E) bicarbonate

7. If the extracellular concentration of a substance doubles from 10 mM to 20 mM while the intracellular concentration remains at 5 mM, the rate of diffusion increases

(A) twofold
(B) threefold
(C) fourfold
(D) fivefold
(E) tenfold

8. Which of the following statements best characterizes a molecule whose reflection coefficient to a membrane is zero?

(A) It will not permeate the membrane
(B) It can only cross the membrane through the lipid bilayer
(C) It causes water to flow across the membrane
(D) It is as diffusible through the membrane as water
(E) It is transported across the membrane by a carrier

9. The characteristic of a water-insoluble substance most important in governing its diffusibility through a cell membrane is its

(A) hydrated diameter
(B) molecular weight
(C) electrical charge
(D) lipid solubility
(E) three-dimensional shape

10. Which one of the following muscle proteins plays an important role in contraction of both smooth and striated muscle?

(A) Calmodulin
(B) Troponin
(C) Tropomyosin
(D) Actin
(E) Myosin light chains

11. During the process of excitation-contraction coupling in smooth muscle, calcium is released from the sarcoplasmic reticulum by

(A) inositol triphosphate (IP$_3$)
(B) protein kinase C
(C) diacyl glycerol (DAG)
(D) cyclic AMP (cAMP)
(E) calmodulin

12. Which of the following words or phrases is most closely associated with an end-plate potential at the neuromuscular junction?

(A) "All-or-none response"
(B) Depolarization
(C) Hyperpolarization
(D) Membrane propagation
(E) Electrically excitable gates

13. In a nerve, the magnitude of the action potential overshoot is normally a function of the

(A) magnitude of the stimulus
(B) intracellular potassium concentration
(C) extracellular sodium concentration
(D) resting membrane potential
(E) diameter of the axon

14. When circulating catecholamines bind to beta receptors on bronchiolar smooth muscle, their primary effect is caused by the

(A) opening of receptor-activated calcium channels
(B) release of calcium from the sarcoplasmic reticulum
(C) phosphorylation of intracellular proteins
(D) depolarization of the cell membrane
(E) activation of troponin C

15. Which of the following is an important component of excitation-contraction coupling in both smooth and skeletal muscle?

(A) The inward flow of calcium across the muscle membrane
(B) The binding of myosin cross-bridges to actin filaments
(C) The binding of calcium to troponin
(D) The phosphorylation of myosin
(E) The depolarization of the muscle membrane

16. Which of the following statements about impulse transmission at the myoneural junction is true?

(A) It is enhanced by high levels of cholinesterase
(B) It is associated with an influx of potassium ions through the muscle membrane
(C) It is depressed by abnormally low levels of magnesium
(D) It is unaffected by extremely high rates of stimulation of the nerve fiber
(E) It is dependent on the release of acetylcholine from the α motoneuron

17. When comparing the contractile responses in smooth and skeletal muscle, which of the following factors is most different?

(A) The source of activator calcium
(B) The role of calcium in initiating contraction
(C) The mechanism of force generation
(D) The source of energy used during contraction
(E) The nature of the contractile proteins

18. The amount of tension that a whole muscle can produce is greatest in which of the following situations?

(A) In the single twitch response
(B) When extracellular Ca^{2+} is decreased
(C) When extracellular Mg^{2+} is increased
(D) During maximal complete tetanus
(E) When all the fibers are excited by a single stimulus pulse

19. The velocity of nerve conduction is increased with a decrease in the

(A) diameter of the nerve fiber
(B) degree of myelinization
(C) space constant of the nerve fiber
(D) capacitance of the nerve fiber membrane
(E) resting membrane potential

20. The rate of diffusion of a particle across a membrane will increase if

(A) the area of the membrane decreases
(B) the thickness of the membrane increases
(C) the size of the particle increases
(D) the concentration gradient of the particle decreases
(E) the lipid solubility of the particle increases

21. Simple and facilitated diffusion are alike in that both

(A) display saturation kinetics
(B) require some sort of carrier mechanism for transport
(C) can work in the absence of ATP
(D) can transport material against a concentration gradient
(E) can be blocked by specific inhibitors

22. The flow of calcium into the cell is an important component of the upstroke phase of action potentials in

(A) cardiac ventricular muscle
(B) intestinal smooth muscle
(C) skeletal muscle fibers
(D) nerve cell bodies
(E) none of the above

23. The membrane potential will depolarize by the greatest amount if the membrane permeability increases for

(A) potassium
(B) sodium and potassium
(C) chloride
(D) potassium and chloride
(E) sodium, potassium, and chloride

24. Which of the following will be less during the overshoot of an action potential than during the resting state?

(A) Membrane conductance for sodium
(B) Membrane conductance for potassium
(C) Transference for sodium
(D) Transference for potassium
(E) Total membrane conductance

25. If the membrane conductances for sodium and potassium are equal, the membrane potential is close to

(A) -90 mV
(B) -70 mV
(C) -15 mV
(D) 0 mV
(E) $+40$ mV

26. Statements descriptive of both the equilibrium and steady states include which of the following?

(A) The sum of all the fluxes across the membrane is zero in both
(B) Both are maintained by the consumption of free energy
(C) The concentration gradient across the membrane is zero in both
(D) Both are maintained by homeostatic processes
(E) The membrane potential is zero in both

27. During the relative refractory period

(A) the rate of depolarization is decreased
(B) the rate of repolarization is increased
(C) the threshold for eliciting an action potential is decreased
(D) the conductance of potassium is decreased
(E) the magnitude of the overshoot is increased

28. An increase in sodium conductance is associated with

(A) the plateau phase of the ventricular muscle action potential
(B) the downstroke of the skeletal muscle action potential
(C) the upstroke of the smooth muscle action potential
(D) the refractory period of the nerve cell action potential
(E) the end-plate potential of the skeletal muscle fiber

29. Electrically excitable gates are normally involved in

(A) the depolarization of the end-plate membrane by ACh
(B) hyperpolarization of the rods by light
(C) release of calcium from ventricular muscle sarcoplasmic reticulum
(D) transport of glucose into cells by a sodium-dependent, secondary active transport system
(E) increase in nerve cell potassium conductance caused by an increase in extracellular potassium

30. The sodium gradient across the nerve cell membrane is

(A) a result of the Donnan equilibrium
(B) significantly changed during an action potential
(C) used as a source of energy for the transport of other ions
(D) an important determinant of the resting membrane potential
(E) maintained by an Na-Ca exchanger

31. Increasing the extracellular potassium concentration will

(A) increase the threshold for eliciting an action potential
(B) hyperpolarize the membrane potential
(C) decrease potassium permeability
(D) decrease the activity of the sodium-potassium pump
(E) do none of the above

32. Which of the following would cause an immediate reduction in the amount of potassium leaking out of a cell?

(A) Increasing the permeability of the membrane to potassium
(B) Increasing the intracellular potassium concentration
(C) Increasing (hyperpolarizing) the membrane potential
(D) Reducing the activity of the sodium-potassium pump
(E) Decreasing the potassium equilibrium potential

33. Excitation-contraction coupling in smooth muscle is initiated when calcium binds to

(A) myosin light chains
(B) calmodulin
(C) troponin
(D) tropomyosin
(E) protein kinase A

DIRECTIONS: Each numbered question or incomplete statement below is NEGATIVELY phrased. Select the **one best** lettered response.

34. Excitation-contraction coupling in skeletal muscle involves all the following events EXCEPT

(A) generation of end-plate potential
(B) binding of Ca^{2+} to myosin
(C) formation of cross-linkages between actin and myosin
(D) depolarization along transverse tubules
(E) hydrolysis of ATP to ADP

35. Correct comparisons between fast- and slow-twitch skeletal muscle fibers include all the following EXCEPT

(A) fast-twitch fibers fatigue more rapidly
(B) fast-twitch fibers develop more force
(C) fast-twitch fibers store more glycogen
(D) fast-twitch fibers require a higher frequency of stimulation to produce tetanus
(E) fast-twitch fibers contain a higher concentration of mitochondria

36. The flow of water in an osmotic pressure gradient is correctly described by all the following statements EXCEPT

(A) there is a net flow of water from a region of low osmotic pressure to one of a higher osmotic pressure
(B) the rate of water flow increases as the hydraulic conductivity of the membrane increases
(C) there is a net flow of water from a region of low concentration of solute to a region of highly concentrated solute
(D) the rate of water flow increases as the reflection coefficient increases
(E) free energy is required for the flow of water

37. All the following transport processes require energy EXCEPT the movement of

(A) sodium out of nerve cells
(B) calcium into the sarcoplasmic reticulum
(C) hydrogen into the lumen of the distal nephron
(D) glucose into adipose tissue
(E) potassium into striated muscle cells

DIRECTIONS: Each group of questions below consists of lettered headings followed by a set of numbered items. For each numbered item select the **one** lettered heading with which it is **most** closely associated. Each lettered heading may be used **once, more than once, or not at all**.

Questions 38–39

Match each of the descriptions to one of the points on the action potential diagrammed below.

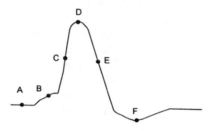

38. Sodium current exceeds potassium current

39. The driving force for sodium is greatest

Questions 40–42

Match each action to the protein with which it is most closely associated.

(A) Calmodulin
(B) Troponin
(C) Tropomyosin
(D) Myosin
(E) Myosin light chain kinase
(F) Phospholamban
(G) Protein kinase A
(H) Actin
(I) Phospholipase C

40. Binds to calcium during smooth muscle excitation-contraction coupling

41. Regulates the activity of the calcium pump on the sarcoplasmic reticulum

42. Activated by epinephrine via a G-protein–mediated process

Questions 43–44

Match each of the actions listed below to one of the synaptic transmitters.

(A) γ-Aminobutyric acid (GABA)
(B) Acetylcholine (ACh)
(C) Norepinephrine
(D) Glutamate
(E) Nitric oxide

43. Opens a chloride channel

44. Opens the NMDA channel

Cellular Physiology
Answers

1.   The answer is C. *(West, 12/e, pp 41–45.)* The conduction velocity of an action potential along an axon is proportional to the axon's diameter for both unmyelinated and myelinated axons. In myelinated axons, the conduction velocity of an action potential also increases as the distance between nodes of Ranvier increases. The resting potential and the action potential of a nerve axon are dependent on the type and density of electrically excitable gates and the ability of the Na,K-ATPase to establish and maintain the concentration gradients. These characteristics are not related in any systematic way to the axon diameter.

2.   The answer is B. *(Berne, 3/e, pp 10–13.)* When the intracellular and extracellular solute concentrations of a cell are different from each other, water will flow across the cell membrane at a rate proportional to the osmotic pressure difference. However, the new steady-state volume of the cell will depend only on the difference between the concentration of solutes that are not permeable to the cell. Solute that is permeable to the cell will eventually reach diffusional equilibrium and will have no effect on the eventual volume of the cell. Sodium chloride, glucose, and $CaCl_2$ all behave as if they were impermeable to the cell membrane, and thus all will contribute to the steady-state change in volume caused by the osmotic flow of water. The osmolarity of the 200 mM solution of NaCl is 400 mOsm and is the highest of the solutions containing nonpermeable solute. A solution containing a concentration of impermeable solutes that is higher than the solute concentration of a normal cell (i.e., greater than 280 to 290 mOsm) is called a *hypertonic* solution; a solution with a concentration of impermeable solutes that is less than that of a normal cell is called a *hypotonic* solution.

3.   The answer is C. *(Berne, 3/e, pp 33–35, 49.)* Increasing the extracellular concentration of K^+ causes the cell to depolarize, that is, to become more positive. When the cell depolarizes, the activation gate on the K^+ channel opens, causing K^+ conductance to rise. Depolarization also causes the activation gate (the m gate) on the Na^+ channel to open and the inactivation gate (the h gate) to close. As a result, Na^+ conductance remains the same. However, because many of the Na^+ channels are inactivated, the cell becomes less excitable. The activity of the Na-K pump will decrease if K^+ concentration is decreased.

4. The answer is C. *(Berne, 3/e, pp 748–749, 795–797.)* Secondary active transport processes typically use the energy contained in the Na^+ concentration gradient to carry material across the membrane against their concentration gradients. The reabsorption of HPO_4^{2-} by the renal proximal tubule is accomplished by a secondary active transport process. Two Na^+ ions are used by the carrier, making the process electrically neutral. The secretion of H^+ by the distal tubule, the reabsorption of Ca^{2+} by the sarcoplasmic reticulum (SR), and the removal of Na^+ from a nerve axon all involve a primary active transport system in which the energy obtained from the hydrolysis of ATP is directly used to transport the material across the membrane. K^+ flows passively out of a cardiac myocyte.

5. The answer is D. *(Berne, 3/e, pp 58–59.)* Membrane excitability is related to the ease with which Na^+ channels open when the cell is depolarized. The activation of Na^+ channels or the opening of the m gate is governed in part by the extracellular Ca^{2+} concentration. When extracellular Ca^{2+} is lowered, the m gate can open at more negative membrane potentials, and therefore the membrane is more easily excitable. Although increasing extracellular K^+ will bring the membrane closer to threshold and thus may make it more excitable, its predominant effect is to cause the inactivation of Na^+ channels by the closing of the h gates. Inactivation of sodium channels makes the cell membrane less excitable.

6. The answer is A. *(West, 12/e, pp 36–38.)* The membrane potential is determined by the concentration gradient of the ion to which it is most permeable or for which it has the greatest conductance. In the resting state, the conductance for potassium is approximately nine times as great as the conductance for sodium. Hence, the membrane potential is dependent on the concentration gradient for potassium. The concentration gradient for chloride is not an important determinant of the membrane potential (even in those cells where chloride conductance is high) because, unlike sodium and potassium, which are actively pumped across the membrane, chloride is passively distributed across the membrane.

7. The answer is B. *(Guyton, 8/e, pp 43–44.)* According to Fick's law of diffusion, the rate of diffusion (flux) is proportional to the difference in concentration between the inside (Cin) and outside (Cout) of the membrane: Flux = P (Cin − Cout). In the example given, initially this difference was 10 mM − 5 mM, or 5 mM. With the change in extracellular concentration, the difference became 20 mM − 5 mM, or 15 mM. Since the concentration difference increased threefold (from 5 to 15), the rate of diffusion also increased threefold.

8. The answer is D. *(Berne, 3/e, pp 8–12.)* The reflection coefficient is a measure of a membrane's permeability to a substance in comparison to its permeability in water. It can be calculated from the following equation:

$$\text{Reflection coefficient} = \frac{P\,(\text{water}) - P\,(\text{substance})}{P\,(\text{water})}$$

It is also a measure of the actual osmotic pressure developed by the substance compared with the osmotic pressure it should theoretically develop according to Van't Hoff's equation. A substance with a reflection coefficient of zero would have the same diffusibility through the membrane as water and would not develop any osmotic pressure.

9. The answer is D. *(Berne, 3/e, pp 7–10.)* Materials that are not soluble in water can only cross the membrane through the lipid bilayer. The most important factor determining how well a substance can diffuse across the lipid bilayer is the substance's lipid solubility. If two materials have the same lipid solubility, then the diffusion coefficient of the smaller particle will be greater.

10. The answer is D. *(Berne, 3/e, pp 294–296, 316–322, 399–403.)* In excitation-contraction coupling in striated muscle, calcium initiates contraction by binding to troponin. The calcium-activated troponin then acts to remove the tropomyosin-mediated inhibition of actin-myosin interaction. In excitation-contraction coupling in smooth muscle, calcium initiates contraction by binding to calmodulin. The calcium-activated calmodulin then acts as a protein kinase, phosphorylating the myosin light chains. Actin-myosin interaction follows light-chain phosphorylation. In both smooth and striated muscle, the thin filaments are composed of actin.

11. The answer is A. *(Berne, 3/e, pp 320–321.)* The release of calcium from the sarcoplasmic reticulum in many smooth muscles is mediated by IP_3. When a calcium-mobilizing stimulus binds to its receptor on the cell membrane, it activates a phosphatase enzyme, phospholipase C. The phospholipase C cleaves inositol diphosphate (a membrane-bound lipid) into IP_3 and DAG. IP_3 causes the release of calcium from the sarcoplasmic reticulum. DAG activates protein kinase C, whose function is not well understood.

12. The answer is B. *(Guyton, 8/e, pp 81–83.)* An end-plate potential is a depolarization caused by the opening of chemically excitable gates in response to the release of acetylcholine from the presynaptic nerve terminals of alpha motoneurons. Its magnitude is proportional to the amount of transmitter released. Although it is not propagated, it acts as a stimulus for the generation of an action potential on the muscle membrane contiguous to the end-plate region. The action potential is propagated and results in a muscle twitch.

13. The answer is C. *(Guyton, 8/e, pp 55–58.)* An action potential is normally an all-or-none response; that is, its magnitude is independent of the stimulus strength. The magnitude of the action potential is reduced during the relative refractory period or when the membrane is depolarized by an abnormally high extracellular potassium concentration. However, the upstroke of the action potential is caused by an inward flow of sodium ions, and thus its magnitude depends on the extracellular sodium concentration.

14. The answer is C. *(Berne, 3/e, pp 77–79, 81–83.)* When norepinephrine, epinephrine, or exogenously administered catecholamines bind to beta receptors, they activate a guanyl nucleotide-binding protein called the G_s (or N_s) protein. The activated G protein in turn activates adenylate cyclase, which catalyzes the conversion of ATP into cyclic AMP (cAMP). The cAMP then activates a protein kinase (cAMP-dependent protein kinase). The protein kinase phosphorylates a variety of intracellular and membrane proteins that produce the relaxation of bronchiolar smooth muscle observed in response to adrenergic agonist stimulation.

15. The answer is B. *(Berne, 3/e, pp 294–296, 316–322, 478–480. Ganong, 16/e, p 61.)* Excitation-contraction coupling in skeletal muscle requires membrane depolarization and the binding of calcium to troponin. In contrast, smooth muscle can contract in the absence of membrane depolarization (by a process called *pharmacomechanical coupling*) and does not contain troponin. Smooth muscle contraction is initiated by cross-bridge phosphorylation. In skeletal muscle calcium is derived exclusively from the sarcoplasmic reticulum, whereas in smooth muscle a significant portion of the calcium comes from the extracellular fluid. Contraction in both is due to the sliding of the thin (actin) filaments across the thick (myosin) filaments brought about by the binding of myosin cross-bridges to the actin filaments.

16. The answer is E. *(West, 12/e, pp 59–60.)* Impulse transmission at the myoneural junction depends on the release of acetylcholine. High levels of cholinesterase would tend to interfere with transmission, as would high (not low) levels of magnesium. The release of acetylcholine at the myoneural junction is thought to be associated with an influx of calcium ions into the terminal membranes. Extremely rapid rates of stimulation cause depletion of acetylcholine stores and would result in fatigue of the myoneural junction.

17. The answer is B. *(Berne, 3/e, pp 294–296, 316–322.)* In both smooth and skeletal muscle, force is generated by the cycling of cross-bridges. ATP provides the energy for the cycling of the cross-bridges in both muscles. In skeletal muscle, activator calcium comes exclusively from the sarcoplasmic reticulum (SR), while in smooth muscle calcium can come both from the SR and from the extracellular fluid. However, the greatest difference in excitation-contraction coupling involves the role of calcium in initiating contraction. In smooth muscle, calcium binds to and activates calmodulin, which acts as a kinase to catalyze the phosphorylation of the 20,000-dalton myosin light chain (LC$_{20}$). Once the light chains are phosphorylated, myosin cross-bridges bind to actin on the thin filaments, which initiates contraction. In skeletal muscle, calcium binds to troponin, which removes the tropomyosin-mediated inhibition of the actin-myosin interactions. Once the inhibition is removed, cross-bridge cycling (and contraction) begins.

18. The answer is D. *(Berne, 3/e, pp 294–296. Guyton, 8/e, pp 74–76.)* The single muscle twitch generates only a single, sudden contraction. During summation, individual muscle twitches are added together to make strong muscle movements. Indeed, the tension developed during summation is much greater than during the single muscle twitch. When a muscle is stimulated at progressively greater frequencies, activation of the contractile mechanism occurs repeatedly before any relaxation has occurred and the successive contractions fuse into one continuous contraction. Such a response is called *tetanus*. During complete tetanus there is no relaxation between stimuli; during incomplete tetanus there are periods of incomplete relaxation between the summated stimuli. The tension developed during complete tetanus is about four times that developed by the individual twitch contractions.

19. The answer is D. *(Berne, 3/e, pp 50–53.)* In order for propagation of an action potential to occur the depolarization produced by one action potential must depolarize the adjacent patch of excitable membrane to threshold. The amount of charge that must flow to produce this depolarization varies inversely with the membrane capacitance. Thus, as the capacitance decreases, the velocity of conduction increases. The rate of charge flow decreases as the diameter of the nerve fiber decreases, thus decreasing the velocity of conduction. The space constant ($\sqrt{R_m/R_{in}}$) is a measure of how far along the axon the charge will flow. The degree of myelinization determines the magnitude of the membrane resistance (R_m); thus, when myelinization decreases, membrane resistance decreases and the space constant decreases. Velocity of conduction decreases as the space constant decreases. Decreasing the resting membrane potential inactivates sodium channels. This will decrease the flow of charge across the membrane during an action potential and thus decrease the velocity of propagation.

20. The answer is E. *(West, 12/e, pp 17–19.)* The rate of diffusion is described by Fick's law, which states that the flux of material across a membrane is directly proportional to the area of a membrane and the concentration difference of the particles on either side of the membrane and is inversely proportional to the thickness of the membrane. In general, if all other properties of the membrane are the same, the larger the particle the more difficulty it will have crossing the membrane. Similarly, for a particle to cross a membrane, it must first dissolve in the membrane. For lipid-soluble substances, the greater the lipid solubility, the greater the amount dissolved in the membrane and the greater the flux.

21. The answer is C. *(West, 12/e, pp 17–19, 21–22.)* Neither simple nor facilitated diffusion requires free energy to transport material across a membrane, so both can function in the absence of ATP. Because they do not use free energy, neither can transport material against a concentration gradient. Facilitated diffusion is a carrier-mediated process and so displays saturation kinetics and can be blocked by specific inhibitory substances that bind to the carrier.

22. The answer is B. *(Berne, 3/e, pp 36, 39–40, 47–48.)* In cells of the cardiac ventricular muscle, the plateau phase of the action potential, but not the upstroke, is accompanied by the flow of calcium into the cells. In intestinal smooth muscle, the upstroke of the action potential is caused by the flow of calcium into the cell. Skeletal muscle fibers resemble nerve fibers. In both of these cells, the upstroke of the action potential is caused by the flow of sodium into the cell.

23. The answer is B. *(West, 12/e, pp 35–38.)* When the permeability of a particular ion is increased, the membrane potential moves toward the equilibrium potential for that ion. The equilibrium potentials for chloride (-80mV) and potassium (-92 mV) are close to the resting membrane potential, so increases in their permeability have little effect on the resting membrane potential. The equilibrium potential for sodium ($+60$mV) is very far from the resting membrane potential. Thus, increasing the permeability for sodium causes a large depolarization. When the increase in sodium permeability is combined with an increase in potassium permeability, the amount of depolarization produced is greater than that produced when sodium, potassium, and chloride permeabilities are all increased.

24. The answer is D. *(West, 12/e, pp 35–38, 47–51.)* During an action potential the conductance for both sodium and potassium is higher than it is at rest. However, the conductance for sodium is higher than the conductance for potassium during the overshoot. Hence, the transference for potassium is less. Recall that transference is a measure of an ion's relative conductance:

$$\text{Transference (ion)} = \frac{\text{Conductance (ion)}}{\text{Total conductance}}$$

25. The answer is C. *(West, 12/e, pp 37–38.)* The membrane potential can be calculated using the equivalent circuit analysis based on the principle that the net current flow through the membrane at rest is zero. According to the equivalent circuit analysis, $E_m =$

$$\frac{(E_K \times g_K) + (E_{Na} \times g_{Na})}{g_K + g_{Na}}$$

Solving this equation when $g_K = g_{Na}$ yields

$$\frac{-92 + +60}{2} = -16\,\text{mV}$$

26. The answer is A. *(West, 12/e, pp 14–18, 28–30.)* In both an equilibrium and a steady state condition, there is no change in the concentration of materials inside or outside the cell. However, in a steady state condition energy must be consumed to keep the concentrations from changing. An equilibrium condition is not considered to be a homeostatic process because active physiologic mechanisms are not used to maintain it. Membrane potential and concentration differences across the membrane can be maintained in both states.

27. The answer is A. *(Berne, 3/e, pp 48–49. Guyton, 8/e, p 64.)* During the relative refractory period, an action potential can still be elicited, but the stimulus must be stronger than normal. The larger stimulus is required because the threshold is increased owing to the increases in potassium conductance and sodium inactivation that occur during the action potential. These changes in membrane permeability are also responsible for causing the decreases in the rate of rise and overshoot of the action potential that occur during the relative refractory period. The decrease in the overshoot potential causes a decrease in the number of potassium channels that open during the action potential. Thus the repolarization phase of the action potential is slower than normal.

28. The answer is E. *(Berne, 3/e, pp 36, 39–40, 47–48, 58–59.)* The channel opened by ACh when it binds to receptors on the end plates of skeletal muscle fibers is equally permeable to potassium and sodium. The increase in sodium permeability allows sodium to flow into the cell and produces the end-plate potential. The plateau phase of ventricular muscle action potentials and the upstroke of smooth muscle action potentials are produced by an increase in calcium conductance. An increase in potassium conductance is responsible for the downstroke of the action potential. The refractory period is caused by an increase in potassium conductance and a decrease in the number of sodium channels available to produce an action potential (i.e., sodium channel inactivation).

29. The answer is E. *(Berne, 3/e, pp 21–23, 58–59, 151–152, 399–403.)* Electrically excitable gates are those that respond to a change in membrane potential. The most notable electrically excitable gates are those on the sodium and potassium channels that produce the nerve action potential. The potassium channel gate is opened by depolarization. When potassium is added to the extracellular fluid, it depolarizes the nerve cell membrane and causes the electrically excitable gates on the potassium channel to open. Ventricular muscle sarcoplasmic reticulum releases its calcium in response to an increase in intracellular calcium. In skeletal muscle, depolarization of the T tubule causes electrically driven calcium channels on the SR to open. The gates opened by ACh are chemically excitable gates. In rods, sodium channels are closed when cGMP is hydrolyzed. Glucose transport is not regulated by gates.

30. The answer is C. *(Berne, 3/e, pp 15–17, 19–21, 29–34.)* The sodium-potassium pump uses the energy contained in ATP to maintain the sodium gradient across the membrane. The sodium gradient, in turn, is used to transport other substances across the membrane. For example, the Na-Ca exchanger uses the energy in the sodium gradient to help maintain the low intracellular calcium required for normal cell function. Although sodium enters the cell during an action potential, the quantity of sodium is so small that no significant change in intracellular sodium concentration occurs. Because the sodium transference is so low, the sodium equilibrium potential is not an important determinant of the resting membrane potential.

31. The answer is A. *(Berne, 3/e, pp 39–43, 49, 368–370.)* When the extracellular potassium concentration is increased, the membrane depolarizes. Depolarization causes potassium channels to open, which increases potassium permeability. Depolarization also causes sodium channels to inactivate, which reduces the number of sodium channels that are able to open in response to a stimulus. Since fewer channels can respond to the stimulus, a larger-than-normal stimulus is required to generate an action potential. The activity of the sodium-potassium pump may increase somewhat in response to the increase in extracellular potassium. However, the increase will be quite small because the potassium binding sites on the pump are nearly saturated at normal physiologic potassium concentrations.

32. The answer is C. *(Berne, 3/e, pp 31–34.)* The amount of potassium leaking out of the cell depends on its driving force and its membrane conductance. The driving force is the difference between the membrane potential and the equilibrium potential for potassium. Since the membrane potential is more positive than the equilibrium potential for potassium, hyperpolarizing the membrane (that is, making it more negative) would reduce the driving force. Increasing the intracellular potassium concentration increases the equilibrium potential for potassium, that is, makes it more negative and thus increases the driving force. Reducing the sodium-potassium pump activity would cause the potassium concentration gradient to fall, which, in turn, would cause a decrease in the amount of potassium leaking out of the cell. However, this would not occur immediately. In fact, because the pump is electrogenic, a small depolarization would initially follow a cessation of pump activity and this would cause an increase in the driving force for potassium.

33. The answer is B. *(Berne, 3/e, pp 316–319.)* Smooth muscle contraction is regulated by a series of reactions that begins with the binding of calcium to calmodulin. The calcium-calmodulin complex then binds to and activates a protein kinase called *myosin light chain kinase (MLCK)*. MLCK catalyzes the phosphorylation of the myosin light chains (LC_{20}). Once these light chains are phosphorylated, myosin and actin interaction can occur and the muscle shortens and develops tension. Although two molecules of ATP are required to initiate contraction, one for the phosphorylation of myosin light chains and one to bend the myosin cross-bridge, smooth muscle is energetically efficient because the rate of cross-bridge cycling is so slow.

34. The answer is B. *(Berne, 3/e, pp 294–296.)* In excitation-contraction coupling, depolarization of the muscle fiber follows generation of the end-plate potential. The depolarization is transmitted via the transverse tubule system into the inner portion of the muscle fiber, where it triggers release of calcium from sarcoplasmic reticulum. Calcium binds to troponin C, which permits formation of cross-linkages between actin and myosin and sliding of thin and thick filaments. Reaccumulation of calcium by sarcoplasmic reticulum followed by release of calcium from troponin results in cessation of actin-myosin interaction and relaxation.

35. The answer is E. *(Berne, 3/e, pp 298–299.)* Fast-twitch fibers are characterized by their large size, high capacity for anaerobic metabolism, high development of force, high speed of contraction, and short twitch times. They are unable to replenish their ATP supply quickly because they are relatively poorly perfused and have few mitochondria; this results in rapid fatigue. They are able to sustain contraction for a short time because of their relatively large (compared with those of slow-twitch fibers) glycogen stores. They have a short duration of contraction because their SR calcium pumps rapidly resequester calcium. In order for summation or tetanus to occur, a second stimulus must be applied before the muscle relaxes. The shorter the duration of contraction, the more frequently the muscle must be stimulated to produce tetanus.

36. The answer is E. *(Berne, 3/e, pp 10–13.)* The ability of dissolved particles to cause the flow of water across a membrane by osmosis increases when the permeability of the membrane to the particles decreases and increases when the hydraulic conductivity of the membrane to water increases. An increase in the reflection coefficient indicates that the permeability of the membrane to the particles is decreasing. The osmotic pressure is higher on the side of the membrane where the concentration of particles is higher, but, paradoxically, the osmotic flow of water is toward the side of the membrane that has the higher osmotic pressure.

37. The answer is D. *(Berne, 3/e, pp 13–25.)* Glucose is transported into fat cells by facilitated diffusion and thus does not require the direct or indirect use of energy. Insulin increases the rate of diffusion but is not necessary for the diffusion. Sodium and potassium are transported by the Na-K pump, calcium is transported into the sarcoplasmic reticulum by a Ca pump, and hydrogen is transported by an H^+ pump. All of these transporters use ATP directly in the transport process. In the proximal tubule, hydrogen is secreted by an Na-H exchange process; this is an example of secondary active transport.

38–39. The answers are 38–C, 39–F. *(Berne, 3/e, pp 33–34, 39–42.)* The upstroke of the action potential is caused by the opening of Na^+ channels and the flow of Na^+ into the cell. Depolarization occurs because the Na^+ current exceeds the K^+ current (point C). Until threshold (point B) is reached, however, the Na^+ conductance does not change, and since its driving force ($E_M - E_{Na^+}$) is decreasing during this time, the Na^+ current actually falls while the membrane is being depolarized to threshold.

The maximum driving force for Na^+ is greatest when the membrane is furthest from the E_{Na^+}, that is, at the peak of the undershoot (point F). Potassium current exceeds Na^+ current during the downstroke and is equal to Na^+ current during the resting state (point A), at threshold (point B), and at the peak of the overshoot (point D).

40–42. The answers are 40–A, 41–F, 42–I. *(Berne, 3/e, pp 316–319, 402–403, 821–825.)* When Ca^{2+} binds to calmodulin, the Ca^{2+}-calmodulin complex activates myosin light chain kinase (MLCK), which catalyzes the phosphorylation of the myosin 20-kilodalton light chain (LC_{20}). Once the myosin light chains are phosphorylated, cross-bridge cycling begins and the smooth muscle develops force and shortens.

When not phosphorylated, phospholamban inhibits the activity of the Ca^{2+} pump on the sarcoplasmic reticulum of cardiac and smooth muscle. The phosphorylation of phospholamban is catalyzed by cAMP-dependent protein kinase (protein kinase A). Once phosphorylated, the inhibitory effect of phospholamban is reduced and the activity of the sarcoplasmic reticulum Ca^{2+} pump is increased. The increased sequestering of Ca^{2+} results in the shortening of ventricular contraction in cardiac muscle and the relaxation of smooth muscle.

When epinephrine binds to an α receptor, it activates a G protein that, in turn, activates phospholipase C. Phospholipase C catalyzes the breakdown of phosphatidyl diphosphate (PIP_2) to IP_3 and diacylglycerol (DAG). IP_3 causes the release of Ca^{2+} from the sarcoplasmic reticulum and leads to the contraction of smooth muscle. When epinephrine binds to a β receptor, it activates a G protein that, in turn, activates adenyl cyclase. Adenyl cyclase catalyzes the formation of cAMP from ATP; cAMP activates protein kinase A.

43–44. The answers are 43–A, 44–D. *(Ganong, 16/e, pp 73–74, 93–99, 314, 539–540.)* GABA, or γ-aminobutyric acid, is the most common inhibitory neurotransmitter used by the central nervous system. There are two GABA receptors. $GABA_A$ receptors cause the opening of Cl^- channels. $GABA_B$ receptors work by opening K^+ channels, or, when involved in an axoaxonic synapse, they reduce synaptic transmitter release by activating a second messenger system that closes Ca^{2+} channels. The NMDA channel is a large channel permeable to Ca^{2+}, K^+, and Na^+.

When glutamate binds to an NMDA receptor, the NMDA channel may open if the cell has been previously depolarized by some other synaptic input. Norepinephrine binds to α and β receptors. When norepinephrine binds to an α receptor, it starts a process that leads to the generation of IP_3 and the contraction of smooth muscle. When norepinephrine binds to a β receptor, it starts a process that leads to the generation of cAMP and the relaxation of smooth muscle or to an increase in cardiac contractility. ACh binds to nicotinic and muscarinic receptors. When it binds to nicotinic receptors on skeletal muscle, it causes the opening of channels permeable to Na^+ and K^+. When it binds to muscarinic receptors on smooth muscle, it leads to the generation of IP_3 and muscle contraction. Nitric oxide is the endothelial cell–relaxing factor that causes the dilation of smooth muscle surrounding blood vessels.

Cardiac Physiology

DIRECTIONS: Each question below contains five suggested responses. Select the **one best** response to each question.

45. In a test subject, oxygen consumption was measured at 700 mL/min. Pulmonary artery oxygen content was 140 mL per liter of blood and brachial artery oxygen content was 210 mL per liter of blood. Cardiac output was which of the following?

(A) 4.2 L/min
(B) 7.0 L/min
(C) 10.0 L/min
(D) 12.6 L/min
(E) 30.0 L/min

46. Which one of the following is the best index of preload?

(A) Blood volume
(B) Central venous pressure
(C) Pulmonary capillary wedge pressure
(D) Left ventricular end-diastolic volume
(E) Left ventricular end-diastolic pressure

47. Which one of the following is the best index of afterload?

(A) Left ventricular end-diastolic pressure
(B) Left ventricular mean systolic pressure
(C) Pulmonary capillary wedge pressure
(D) Total peripheral resistance
(E) Mean arterial blood pressure

48. The highest blood flow per gram of left ventricular myocardium would occur

(A) when aortic pressure is highest
(B) when left ventricular pressure is highest
(C) at the beginning of isovolumic contraction
(D) at the end of isovolumic contraction
(E) at the beginning of diastole

49. Which of the following is consistent with the ECG tracing shown below?

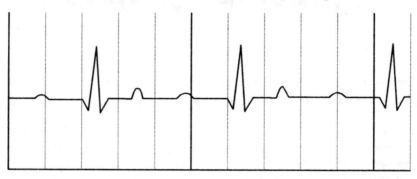

Time (sec)

(A) Bradycardia
(B) First-degree heart block
(C) Second-degree heart block
(D) Third-degree heart block
(E) Tachycardia

50. The mean electrical axis during the ventricular depolarization recorded in the three leads shown below would be closest to

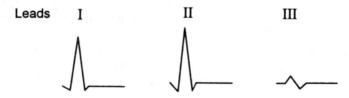

(A) +90 degrees
(B) +60 degrees
(C) +30 degrees
(D) −60 degrees
(E) −90 degrees

51. During ventricular ejection, the pressure difference smallest in magnitude is between the

(A) pulmonary artery and left atrium
(B) right ventricle and right atrium
(C) left ventricle and aorta
(D) left ventricle and left atrium
(E) aorta and capillaries

52. Which of the following would result from a regurgitant aortic valve in a nonfailing heart?

(A) A decrease in diastolic pressure
(B) A decrease in cardiac energy consumption
(C) A systolic murmur
(D) A decrease in heart rate
(E) A decrease in systolic blood pressure

53. Which of the following best describes a second-degree heart block?

(A) The atria fail to activate
(B) Atrial activation is completely dissociated from ventricular activation
(C) The PR interval is prolonged but all the action potentials eventually get through to the ventricles
(D) The PR interval is prolonged and some of the atrial depolarizations are not propagated to the ventricles
(E) Alternate atrial depolarizations are caused by retrograde conduction from the ventricles

54. An increased preload would most likely be caused by an increase in

(A) arteriolar tone
(B) venous tone
(C) myocardial contractility
(D) heart rate
(E) capillary permeability

55. Propagation of the action potential through the heart is slowest in the

(A) atrial muscle
(B) AV node
(C) His bundles
(D) Purkinje fibers
(E) ventricular muscle

56. The greatest benefit derived from administering a positive inotropic drug to a patient in heart failure results from

(A) a reduction in heart rate
(B) a reduction in heart size
(C) an increase in end-diastolic pressure
(D) an increase in wall thickness
(E) an increase in cardiac excitability

57. At which point on the pressure volume curve illustrated below is the afterload on the heart the greatest?

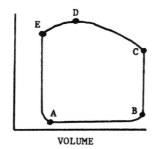

(A) A
(B) B
(C) C
(D) D
(E) E

58. Closure of the aortic valve occurs at the onset of which phase of the cardiac cycle?

(A) Isovolumetric contraction
(B) Rapid ejection
(C) Protodiastole
(D) Isovolumetric relaxation
(E) Rapid filling

59. If the QRS complex is positive in lead II and negative in lead III, the mean electrical axis (MEA) is between

(A) −30 and +30
(B) +30 and +60
(C) +60 and +90
(D) +90 and +120
(E) +120 and +150

60. Persistence of a patent foramen ovale following birth does not cause significant physiologic abnormality because the

(A) left atrial pressure is higher than the right atrial pressure
(B) left ventricular output is greater than the right ventricular output
(C) left ventricular systolic pressure is greater than the right ventricular systolic pressure
(D) closure of the atrioventricular valves precedes ventricular ejection
(E) right atrial systole precedes left atrial systole

61. Splitting of the second heart sound (S_2) into two components is enhanced by

(A) delayed closure of the aortic valve
(B) delayed closure of the mitral valve
(C) early closure of the pulmonic valve
(D) prolongation of atrial systole
(E) none of the above

62. Which of the following statements about the third heart sound (S_3) is correct?

(A) It is usually diminished in congestive heart failure
(B) It is produced by turbulence during rapid ventricular filling in early diastole
(C) It is produced by turbulence following atrial contraction
(D) It is often associated with the "floppy" mitral valve syndrome
(E) It is produced by flow through the patent foramen ovale

63. In a resting, healthy man, the heart pumps how many liters of blood per minute?

(A) 0.9
(B) 2 to 3
(C) 5 to 6
(D) 8 to 10
(E) 15 to 20

64. Sustained elevation of cardiac output will occur with which of the following conditions?

(A) Hypertension
(B) Aortic regurgitation
(C) Anemia
(D) Third-degree heart block
(E) Cardiac tamponade

65. Which of the following will be greater during the plateau phase of the ventricular action potential than at rest?

(A) Sodium conductance
(B) Total membrane conductance
(C) Potassium conductance
(D) Calcium conductance
(E) Chloride conductance

66. Which one of the following statements concerning the mitral valve is correct?

(A) It requires contraction of the papillary muscle in order to initiate closing
(B) A systolic murmur is produced when it fails to close properly
(C) It closes at the end of isovolumic contraction
(D) It normally closes during the PR interval
(E) It prevents backflow of blood into the ventricle during diastole

67. Increasing vagal stimulation of the heart will cause an increase in

(A) heart rate
(B) PR interval
(C) ventricular contractility
(D) ejection fraction
(E) cardiac output

68. During exercise there is an increase in a person's

(A) stroke volume
(B) diastolic pressure
(C) pulmonary arterial pressure
(D) pulmonary arterial resistance
(E) total peripheral resistance

69. If, under resting conditions, the heart rate is 70 beats per minute, the cardiac output is 5.6 L/min, and the end-diastolic volume is 160 mL, what is the ejection fraction?

(A) 0.40
(B) 0.45
(C) 0.50
(D) 0.55
(E) 0.60

70. Phase 4 depolarization of SA nodal cells is caused by

(A) an increase in the flow of sodium into the cell
(B) a decrease in the flow of potassium out of the cell
(C) an increase in the activity of the Na-Ca exchanger
(D) a decrease in the flow of chloride out of the cell
(E) a decrease in the activity of the Na-K pump

71. Cardiovascular changes that occur during inspiration include decreased

(A) right ventricular filling
(B) right ventricular output
(C) pressure gradient from extrathoracic veins to the right atrium
(D) systemic arterial pressure
(E) left ventricular contractility

72. Blood pressure increases and heart rate decreases in response to

(A) exercise
(B) increased body temperature
(C) exposure to high altitude
(D) increased intracranial pressure
(E) hemorrhage

73. During exercise, cardiac output is augmented by

(A) sympathetic stimulation of resistance vessels
(B) dilation of venous vessels
(C) decreased end-diastolic volume
(D) decreased mean systemic arterial pressure
(E) increased ventricular contractility

74. When flow through the mitral valve is restricted by mitral stenosis,

(A) exercise can induce acute pulmonary edema
(B) left ventricular preload increases
(C) left atrial pressure diminishes
(D) right ventricular end-diastolic pressure decreases
(E) central venous pressure decreases

75. Stroke volume can be decreased by

(A) increasing ventricular contractility
(B) increasing heart rate
(C) increasing central venous pressure
(D) decreasing total peripheral resistance
(E) decreasing systemic blood pressure

76. An ectopic extrasystole caused by a ventricular focus is characterized by

(A) interruption of the regular SA node discharge
(B) retrograde conduction of the action potential to the atrium
(C) a skipped ventricular contraction
(D) a skipped atrial contraction
(E) a larger-than-normal force of contraction

DIRECTIONS: Each numbered question or incomplete statement below is NEGATIVELY phrased. Select **one best** lettered response.

77. The electrocardiogram (ECG) is LEAST effective in detecting abnormalities in

(A) the position of the heart in the chest
(B) atrioventricular conduction
(C) cardiac rhythm
(D) cardiac contractility
(E) coronary blood flow

78. Stroke volume will be increased by increasing the contractile activity of all the following EXCEPT

(A) venous vessels
(B) arterial vessels
(C) ventricles
(D) atria
(E) lymphatic vessels

79. All the following would be greater than normal in a person with a dilated failing left ventricle EXCEPT

(A) pulmonary capillary hydrostatic pressure
(B) left ventricular wall tension
(C) left ventricular energy consumption
(D) left ventricular end-diastolic pressure
(E) left ventricular ejection fraction

80. All the following occur during the PR interval EXCEPT

(A) SA nodal depolarization
(B) atrial depolarization
(C) AV nodal depolarization
(D) depolarization of the bundle of His
(E) depolarization of Purkinje fibers

81. An increase in all the following would contribute to an increase in wall stress EXCEPT

(A) end-diastolic volume
(B) transmural pressure across the ventricle
(C) the thickness of the ventricular wall
(D) total peripheral resistance
(E) aortic pressure

82. All the following increase as the heart compensates for aortic regurgitation EXCEPT

(A) left ventricular end-diastolic volume
(B) left ventricular stroke volume
(C) ventricular mass
(D) pulse pressure
(E) net cardiac output

DIRECTIONS: Each group of questions below consists of lettered headings followed by a set of numbered items. For each numbered item select the **one** lettered heading with which it is **most** closely associated. Each lettered heading may be used **once, more than once, or not at all**.

Questions 83–85

The phases of the action potential of ventricular muscle are represented by the lettered points on the diagram. Match each of the events listed below with the phase with which it is most closely associated.

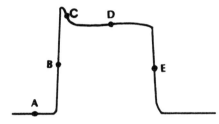

83. An increase in calcium conductance

84. Inactivation of sodium channels

85. Activation of potassium channels

Questions 86–87

Match an interval from the ECG tracing below with each of the events listed.

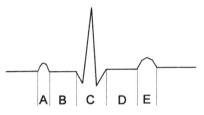

86. Activation of the His bundle

87. Closure of the aortic valve

Questions 88–90

Match one of the points on the left ventricular pressure-volume loop illustrated below to each of the events.

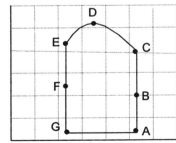

Left Ventricular Volume

88. Isovolumic relaxation

89. Opening of the aortic valve

90. Closure of the mitral valve

Questions 91–94

Match the events in the cardiac cycle with the time points in the pressure tracings below.

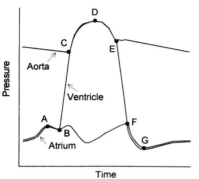

91. Onset of isovolumetric ventricular contraction

92. Closure of aortic valve

93. Opening of mitral valve

94. Completion of atrial systole

Questions 95–98

For each condition listed, select the lettered point on the Frank-Starling curves shown below with which it is most likely to be associated. (Assume point C is the resting state.)

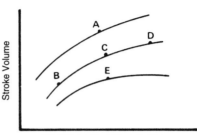

95. Increase in blood volume

96. Myocardial effusion

97. Pericardial effusion

98. Decreased afterload

Questions 99–100

For each circumstance listed below, select the effect on heart rate and blood pressure that is most likely.

(A) Heart rate increased, blood pressure increased

(B) Heart rate increased, blood pressure decreased

(C) Heart rate decreased, blood pressure decreased

(D) Heart rate decreased, blood pressure increased

(E) No change in heart rate and blood pressure

99. Increased intracranial pressure

100. Syncope

Cardiac Physiology
Answers

45. The answer is C. *(Guyton, 8/e, pp 231–232.)* Cardiac output can be measured by using the Fick principle, which asserts that the rate of uptake of a substance by the body (e.g., O_2 consumption in milliliters per minute) is equal to the difference between its concentrations (milliliters per liter of blood) in arterial and venous blood multiplied by the rate of blood flow (cardiac output). This principle is restricted to situations in which arterial blood is the only source of the substance measured. If oxygen consumption by the body at steady state is measured over a period of time and the difference in arterial O_2 and venous O_2 measured by sampling arterial blood and *pulmonary* arterial blood (which is fully mixed venous blood), cardiac output is obtained from the expression

$$\text{cardiac output} = \frac{O_2 \text{ consumption (mL/min)}}{[(A_{O_2}) - (V_{O_2})] \text{ (mL/L)}}$$

Substituting the values for the test subject presented in the question,

$$\text{cardiac output} = \frac{700}{210 - 140} = 10 \text{L/min}$$

46. The answer is D. *(Berne, 3/e, pp 403–404.)* Preload is defined as the sarcomere length at the end of diastole. The parameter most directly related to sarcomere length during this time period is left ventricular end-diastolic volume. Although blood volume, central venous pressure, pulmonary capillary wedge pressure, and left ventricular end-diastolic pressure can all influence preload, they all exert their influence through changes in end-diastolic volume. Each of these parameters could change without altering preload.

47. The answer is B. *(Berne, 3/e, pp 403–404.)* The afterload is the force that the sarcomeres must overcome in order to shorten during systole. According to the law of Laplace, this force is proportional to the pressure (P) and radius (r) of the ventricle during ejection (force $\propto$ P • r). The mean left ventricular systolic pressure would therefore be the best index of afterload. Although total peripheral resistance can influence afterload by causing changes in mean arterial blood pressure, these factors can only influence afterload by causing a change in ventricular pressure. Pulmonary capillary wedge pressure and left ventricular end-diastolic pressure are estimates of the volume of blood in the ventricle during diastole and are indices of preload.

48. The answer is E. *(Berne, 3/e, pp 511–513.)* Blood flow through the coronary vessels of the left ventricle is determined by the ratio of perfusion pressure to vascular resistance. The perfusion pressure is directly related to the aortic pressure at the ostia of the coronaries. Myocardial vascular resistance is significantly influenced by the contractile activity of the ventricle. During systole, when the ventricle is contracting, vascular resistance increases substantially. Flow is highest just at the beginning of diastole because during this phase of the cardiac cycle, aortic pressure is still relatively high and vascular resistance is low due to the fact that the coronary vessels are no longer being squeezed by the contracting myocardium.

49. The answer is B. *(Berne, 3/e, pp 390–391.)* The only abnormality in the ECG illustrated is a prolonged PR interval representing a delay in the propagation of the cardiac action potential from the atria to the ventricles. This is defined as a first-degree heart block. The normal PR interval is between 0.12 and 0.20 s. In a second-degree heart block, some of the P waves are not propagated into the ventricles, but every QRS complex is preceded by a P wave. In third-degree heart block, the atria and ventricles are electrically isolated and thus beat independently. The ventricular rate during a third-degree heart block is typically about 40 beats per minute. Tachycardia is a rapid heart rate above 100 beats per minute, and bradycardia is a slow heart rate below 60 beats per minute. The heart rate from which this ECG tracing was obtained was 75 beats per minute.

50. The answer is C. *(Berne, 3/e, pp 388–390.)* The mean electrical axis (MEA) represents the average direction traveled by the ventricular muscle action potentials as they propagate through the heart. The direction is influenced by the propagation path and the mass of tissue through which the action potentials travel. The MEA is approximately parallel to the axis of the limb lead with the greatest QRS wave magnitude. Since the recording in lead III has no net deflection, the MEA is approximately perpendicular to the axis of this lead. That is, the MEA is perpendicular to the line drawn between +120 degrees and −60 degrees or has a direction of approximately +30 degrees or −150 degrees. Since the QRS wave is positive in leads I and II, the MEA must have the same polarity as these axes and, therefore, must have a positive value. Thus the MEA is approximately +30 degrees.

51. The answer is C. *(West, 12/e, pp 238–243.)* The pressure gradient between regions of the cardiovascular system is directly proportional to the resistance of the intervening structures. During ventricular ejection the aortic valves are open and do not offer any significant resistance to blood flow. Therefore there is very little, if any, pressure difference between the left ventricle and the aorta. Since the tricuspid valve is closed during ventricular ejection, there is an appreciable pressure difference between the right ventricle and the left atrium. Although pulmonary vascular resistance is relatively small compared with systemic vascular resistance, it nonetheless produces a pressure drop between the right ventricle and the left atrium. Since most of the resistance in the systemic vasculature occurs at the level of the arterioles, there is a large pressure gradient between the aorta and the capillaries.

52. The answer is A. *(Guyton, 8/e, pp 257–258.)* Blood leaks from the aorta into the left ventricle during diastole in patients with regurgitant aortic valves. The rapid flow of blood out of the aorta reduces diastolic pressure in the aorta. At the same time, the rapid flow of blood into the left ventricle causes an increase in preload, which results in a larger stroke volume. The large stroke volume injected into the aorta during systole would increase the volume in the arterial system during ejection and therefore increase systolic pressure. The increase in stroke volume would also be associated with an increase in energy consumption by the heart. Murmurs result from the turbulence of blood passing through a narrowed orifice, such as a stenotic valve or one which has not fully closed. Blood flowing from the aorta into the ventricle through the partially opened aortic valve produces the sounds responsible for the diastolic murmur associated with a regurgitant aortic valve. If too much of the stroke volume flows back into the heart during diastole, mean blood pressure will fall and the baroreceptor reflex will cause an increase in heart rate.

53. The answer is D. *(Berne, 3/e, pp 390–391.)* Second-degree heart block is a disturbance in conduction between the atria and the ventricles where some, but not all, of the atrial depolarizations are conducted across the AV node to the ventricles. Therefore, during second-degree heart block, the atrial muscles may depolarize at a normal rhythm but may not always cause the ventricles to beat. On the other hand, when the wave of depolarization passes through the AV node, the ventricles are activated. Therefore, each ventricular beat is preceded by atrial depolarization. Although this is not always true, the propagation through the AV node is often slowed in second-degree heart block and therefore the PR interval is typically prolonged. First-degree heart block is also characterized by a prolongation of the PR interval but differs from second-degree block in that each wave of atrial depolarization propagates into the ventricle. Third-degree heart block is caused by a complete blockage of conduction between the atria and ventricles, and so the beating of the atria and ventricles is completely dissociated. Second-degree heart block is caused by abnormalities in conduction between the atria and ventricles and not by alterations in the rate of phase 4 depolarization.

54. The answer is B. *(Berne, 3/e, pp 499–505.)* Preload is the volume of blood within the ventricles at the end of diastole. Preload can be increased directly by increasing venous volume or decreasing venous capacitance. Thus an increase in venous tone would decrease venous capacitance and lead to an increase in preload. Increasing capillary permeability would decrease vascular blood volume and lead to a decrease in preload. Indirectly, preload can be increased by reducing cardiac output. A reduction in cardiac output leaves a larger portion of the vascular blood volume on the venous side. The increase in venous blood volume leads to a larger preload. Cardiac output is increased by an increase in myocardial contractility and heart rate and so would tend to lower preload. An increase in arteriolar tone, leading to an increase in total peripheral resistance, would tend to trap more blood on the arterial side of the circulation and therefore lower the amount of venous blood. The decrease in venous vascular blood volume would lead to a decrease in preload.

55. The answer is B. *(Berne, 3/e, pp 382–385.)* The propagation of the action potential through the heart is fastest in the His-Purkinje network. The high speed of conduction ensures that the entire ventricle will be depolarized at the same time. The slowest speed of conduction is within the AV node. The delay in propagation between the atria and ventricles provides time for the blood ejected from the atria during atrial systole to enter the ventricles before the ventricles contract.

56. The answer is B. *(West, 12/e, pp 258–259, 307–312.)* The most obvious deleterious effect of a failing heart is the inability to pump enough blood to satisfy the energy requirements of all the tissues. Among the compensatory mechanisms that develop in response to heart failure is an increase in retention of fluid by the kidney. Increased retention of fluid causes the end-diastolic volume of the heart to increase, which, by the Starling mechanism, increases the strength of the heart beat. However, two deleterious effects result from an increase in end-diastolic volume. A larger-than-normal end-diastolic volume causes an increase in end-diastolic pressure, which can lead to pulmonary edema. In addition, the large end-diastolic volume increases the wall stress that must be developed by the heart with each beat, and this increases the myocardial requirement of oxygen. The increase in contractility that results from the administration of a positive inotropic drug such as ouabain will allow the heart to produce the same force at a lower volume and thus eliminate the need for an increase in volume of fluid.

57. The answer is C. *(West, 12/e, pp 223–228.)* Although afterload is sometimes considered equal to the ventricular pressure, wall stress is a truer measure of afterload. Wall stress is proportional to (pressure × radius)/wall thickness. It is greatest at C, where the radius is greater than it is at D. The lower pressure at C does not make up for the greater radius.

58. The answer is D. *(Berne, 3/e, pp 407–412.)* Closure of the semilunar valves (aortic and pulmonic valves) marks the beginning of the isovolumetric relaxation phase of the cardiac cycle. During this brief period (approximately 0.06 s), the ventricles are closed and myocardial relaxation, which began during protodiastole, continues. Intraventricular pressure falls rapidly, although ventricular volume changes little. When intraventricular pressure falls below atrial pressure, the mitral and tricuspid valves open and rapid filling of the ventricles begins.

59. The answer is A. *(Berne, 3/e, pp 387–390.)* If the QRS complex is positive in lead II, the MEA must be between −30 and +120. If the QRS complex is negative in lead III, the MEA must be between −150 and +30. For both conditions to exist, the MEA must be between −30 and +30.

60. The answer is A. *(West, 12/e, pp 903–906.)* In the fetus, the foramen ovale permits most of the oxygenated blood returning to the right atrium to bypass the unoxygenated pulmonary circulation and pass directly into the left atrium, thence into the left ventricle from which the blood is ejected into the systemic circulation via the aorta. The foramen ovale is normally covered by a valvelike leaflet that prevents backflow. At birth, owing to loss of the placental blood flow, there is an increase in systemic vascular resistance, which increases the pressure in the aorta and left atrium, and as the lungs expand there is a decrease in pulmonary vascular resistance, which decreases the pressure in the pulmonary artery and right atrium. Anatomic closure of the foramen ovale prevents left-to-right shunting, although even without closure the pressure gradient between atria is sufficient to keep the valve functionally closed.

61. The answer is E. *(West, 12/e, pp 239–241.)* The second heart sound (S_2) is produced by vibrations in the arterial blood column and arterial walls as the aortic and pulmonic valves undergo tension during closure. Heard over the left sternal border, this sound normally can be resolved into two components representing closure of the aortic and pulmonic valves. Resolution is greatest during inspiration, when venous return increases on the right and prolongs right ventricular ejection. Any event that delays closure of the pulmonic valve thus enhances the splitting; delayed closure of the aortic valve or early closure of the pulmonic valve diminishes the splitting. Closure of the mitral valve and atrial systole influence the first heart sound (S_1).

62. The answer is B. *(West, 12/e, pp 239–241.)* The third heart sound (S_3), also termed the *ventricular diastolic gallop*, is produced by turbulence occurring during the initial phase of rapid ventricular filling in diastole. It may be heard normally in younger persons but is usually louder in patients with congestive heart failure where ventricular compliance is reduced. Turbulence during ventricular filling following atrial contraction at the end of diastole gives rise to the atrial diastolic gallop or fourth heart sound (S_4), also associated with decreased ventricular compliance. Flow through a patent foramen ovale is silent because there is little turbulence in the low-pressure atria.

63. The answer is C. *(Guyton, 8/e, pp 221–223.)* Cardiac output is determined by the product of the stroke volume and heart rate. At rest, stroke volume is about 80 mL and heart rate is 70 beats per minute. Thus, cardiac output would be 5 to 6 L/min in the average healthy man; in the average healthy woman, it is 10 to 20 percent less. Cardiac output can increase several-fold during exercise and would be decreased in the presence of depressed myocardial function and reduced stroke volume, or in the presence of arrhythmias that alter heart rate.

64. The answer is C. *(West, 12/e, pp 315–319.)* The magnitude of the cardiac output is regulated to maintain an adequate blood pressure and to deliver an adequate supply of oxygen to the tissues. In anemia, a greater cardiac output is required to supply oxygen to the tissues because the oxygen-carrying capacity of the blood is reduced. In aortic regurgitation, the stroke volume will be increased. However, a portion of the blood ejected by the heart will return to the heart during diastole. Thus the output delivered to the tissues does not increase despite the fact that the blood ejected by the heart has increased. In hypertension, third-degree heart block, and cardiac tamponade (decreased filling of the heart due to accumulation of fluid within the pericardium), cardiac output will be normal or, if compensation is not possible, cardiac output will be reduced.

65. The answer is D. *(Berne, 3/e, pp 364–375.)* During the plateau phase of the cardiac action potential, potassium conductance decreases below its resting value while calcium conductance is greater than it is at rest. However, the decrease in potassium conductance is greater than the increase in calcium conductance, so total membrane conductance decreases. The sodium channels inactivate during the plateau phase, returning sodium conductance to its resting value.

66. The answer is B. *(West, 12/e, pp 115–117, 239–242.)* The mitral valve is situated between the left ventricle and left atrium and acts to prevent the flow of blood from the ventricle to the atrium during isovolumic contraction. If the valve fails to close properly, blood will flow into the atrium during ventricular contraction and produce a systolic murmur. The valve normally closes at the beginning of isovolumic contraction, which occurs after the QRS complex has begun rather than within the PR interval. Contraction of the papillary muscles pulls on the chordae tendineae, which prevents the mitral valve from being pushed too far into the atrium during ventricular contraction. However, the papillary muscles do not contribute to the closing of the valve.

67. The answer is B. *(Berne, 3/e, pp 417–418.)* The vagal fibers innervating the heart stimulate intracardiac postganglionic fibers, which release acetylcholine (ACh). The postganglionic fibers innervate the SA and AV nodal fibers. ACh causes a decrease in the rate of phase 4 depolarization, thus slowing the heart, and a decrease in conduction velocity through the AV node, thus increasing the PR interval. ACh also causes a slight decrease in contractility. Decreasing the heart rate increases the amount of time available for ventricular filling and thus increases end-diastolic volume. However, the end-systolic volume will be somewhat elevated because of the slight decrease in contractility and increase in afterload. Thus, the ejection fraction will remain the same or decrease slightly.

68. The answer is A. *(West, 12/e, pp 304–306.)* During exercise, increased oxygen consumption and increased venous return to the heart result in an increase in cardiac output and an increase in blood flow to both skeletal muscle and the coronary circulation, where oxygen utilization is greatest. The increase in cardiac output is due to an increase in both heart rate and stroke volume. Systemic arterial pressure also increases in response to the increase in cardiac output. However, the fall in total peripheral resistance, which is caused by dilation of the blood vessels within the exercising muscles, results in a decrease in diastolic pressure. The pulmonary vessels undergo passive dilation as more blood flows into the pulmonary circulation. As a result, pulmonary vascular resistance decreases and pulmonary blood volume increases as cardiac output increases. Pulmonary artery pressure may increase if the increase in cardiac output is unusually large.

69. The answer is C. *(Guyton, 8/e, p 103.)* The ejection fraction is defined as the stroke volume divided by the end-diastolic volume. If the cardiac output is 5.6 L/min and the heart rate is 70 beats per minute, then the stroke volume is 5600/70 = 80 mL. The ejection fraction is thus 80/160 = 0.50.

70. The answer is A. *(Berne, 3/e, pp 378–381.)* Phase 4 depolarization is caused by the activation of two currents: a sodium current and a calcium current. The sodium current is activated when the cell repolarizes. The greater the repolarization, the greater the sodium current. Because of the unusual way in which this current is activated, it is called the *funny current*(i_f). The calcium current is activated near the end of phase 4 depolarization. The calcium current flows through a slowly activated channel and is called the i_{si}. Potassium conductance decreases during phase 4 depolarization and thus the flow of potassium out of the cell is diminished. However, this change in potassium current is not responsible for phase 4 depolarization. Chloride conductance does not change during phase 4. Changes in chloride conductance are not involved in the cardiac action potential. The Na-Ca exchanger maintains low intracellular calcium at rest and may reverse its direction and pump calcium into the cell during phase 2 of the cardiac action potential. However, neither the Na-Ca exchanger nor the Na-K pump is involved in phase 4 depolarization.

71. The answer is D. *(West, 12/e, pp 232–233.)* Because intrathoracic pressure is reduced during inspiration, the pressure gradient from the extrathoracic to intrathoracic veins increases and right ventricular filling and right ventricular output increase. However, pulmonary venous return is decreased by the reduction in intrathoracic pressure. This produces a decrease in *left* ventricular stroke volume, which results in a decrease in systemic arterial pressure.

72. The answer is D. *(Berne, 3/e, pp 523–524, 532–540, 603–604.)* Exercise increases blood pressure and heart rate. Although tissue hypoxia causes arteriolar dilatation, acute hypoxia associated with sudden exposure to high altitudes generates hypertension, as well as excitement, disorientation, and headache. Fever produces tachycardia; blood pressure changes associated with increased body temperature depend on the cause of the temperature. With exercise and increased heat production (and increased blood pressure), vessels dilate in an attempt to dissipate heat. Fever with septic shock will, of course, be associated with a blood pressure decrease owing to vasodilation by endotoxin. Hemorrhage will cause a reflex sympathetic discharge that results in tachycardia and increased total peripheral resistance. If compensation is adequate, blood pressure may not fall. If intracranial pressure is rapidly elevated, cerebral blood flow is reduced. The increase in intracranial pressure stimulates the vasomotor center and produces an increase of systemic blood pressure that may lead to a restoration of cerebral blood flow (Cushing response). A profound bradycardia is also associated with this response.

73. The answer is E. *(Berne, 3/e, pp 532–537.)* During exercise, sympathetic stimulation of the heart and circulating epinephrine cause an increase in ventricular contractility and heart rate leading to an increase in cardiac output. Sympathetic stimulation also causes constriction of the venous vessels, which tends to increase end-diastolic volume. Despite sympathetic stimulation of the resistance vessels, local metabolites produced by the exercising muscles cause small arterioles within the muscles to dilate, which produces a decrease in total peripheral resistance (TPR). However, the fall in TPR does not normally produce a drop in mean systemic blood pressure because the increase in cardiac output is sufficient to counteract the fall in resistance. The increased vascular resistance from sympathetic stimulation of the nonexercising muscles and other organs tends to increase TPR and decrease cardiac output.

74. The answer is A. *(West, 12/e, pp 242, 307.)* In patients with mitral stenosis, the flow of blood from the left atrium to left ventricle during diastole is diminished. The left atrium progressively dilates and left atrial pressure rises. The increase in pressure is transmitted through the pulmonary circulation and eventually leads to an increase in right ventricular pressure. When cardiac output increases during exercise, restriction to flow through the mitral valve causes a sudden increase in pulmonary blood volume, and pulmonary venous and capillary pressures rise, which leads to transudation of fluid into alveoli and pulmonary edema.

75. The answer is B. *(West, 12/e, pp 227–232.)* Stroke volume is determined by preload, afterload, and contractility. Increasing preload by increasing central venous pressure will increase stroke volume. Similarly, decreasing afterload by decreasing total peripheral resistance or systemic blood pressure will cause an increase in stroke volume. Increasing contractility will also increase stroke volume. Cardiac output equals stroke volume times heart rate. If the heart rate increases and cardiac output does not change, stroke volume will decrease.

76. The answer is C. *(Berne, 3/e, pp 390–394.)* A premature heartbeat, or ectopic extrasystole, places the myocardium in a refractory period at the time of arrival of the next normal stimulus from the SA node. Therefore, no ventricular contraction can occur. The impulse from the ectopic focus is incapable of exciting the bundle of His and thus no retrograde conduction to the atrium takes place. Inasmuch as the ectopic event does not extend to the atrium, the atrium continues to contract regularly under the influence of the SA node. The ventricular contraction is smaller because the heart has not filled to its normal end-diastolic volume when the extrasystole occurs. In addition, the extrasystole does not propagate normally through the ventricle so the force of contraction is reduced.

77. The answer is D. *(Berne, 3/e, pp 377–395.)* The ECG records the conduction of the action potential through the heart. Changes in the rate, rhythm, or conduction pathway are recorded. Changes in the position of the heart in the chest will change the size and shape of the ECG recorded by the various leads. Local areas of ischemia caused by changes in coronary blood flow will cause changes in the action potentials that will be reflected in the shape of the ECG recording. The ECG is unable to detect any changes in the ability of the heart to develop force.

78. The answer is B. *(Berne, 3/e, pp 403–404.)* Stroke volume is influenced by ventricular preload, afterload, and contractility. Increasing either ventricular preload or contractility contributes to an increase in stroke volume. Increasing afterload tends to decrease stroke volume. Increasing the contractile activity of the arterial vessels would cause total peripheral resistance to increase, leading to an increase in blood pressure and therefore an increase in afterload. Increasing the contractile activity of the venous vessels, the atria, or the lymphatic vessels could increase the volume of blood entering the left ventricle during diastole and therefore increase stroke volume by increasing preload.

79. The answer is E. *(Guyton, 8/e, pp 245–253.)* When the left ventricle fails, preload is increased as a result of the elevation in left ventricular end-diastolic pressure in an attempt to normalize stroke volume. Since the pulmonary capillaries are supplying the blood to the left ventricle, an increase in left ventricular end-diastolic pressure must be accompanied by an increase in pulmonary capillary hydrostatic pressure. The increase in radius of the dilated ventricle increases wall tension according to the Laplace relationship, $T \propto P \bullet r$ (where T = tension, P = systolic pressure, and r = radius). The increase in wall tension requires an increase in energy consumption. Since the end-diastolic volume increases in order to produce a normal stroke, the ejection fraction (SV/EDV) would be less than normal.

80. The answer is A. *(Berne, 3/e, p 388.)* The PR interval starts at the beginning of the P wave and ends at the beginning of the QRS complex. The physiologic events that occur during this time period include atrial depolarization, which is responsible for the P wave, AV nodal depolarization, and depolarization of the bundle of His and the Purkinje fibers. SA nodal depolarization precedes the P wave. Since the mass of the SA node is so small, this event cannot be detected on the standard ECG recording.

81. The answer is C. *(Berne, 3/e, p 316.)* The factors that influence wall stress are given by the Laplace relationship (WS = [P • r] ÷ Th), where P equals the transmural pressure across the wall of the ventricle, r the radius of the ventricle (determined by end-diastolic volume), and Th the thickness of the ventricular wall. Therefore, increasing the systolic pressure developed by the heart (ventricular transmural pressure) or increasing the end-diastolic volume will increase wall stress. Wall stress will also be increased if total peripheral resistance is increased or aortic pressure is increased because under both conditions, the heart will have to develop more pressure. Wall stress is reduced if the wall thickness increases.

82. The answer is E. *(West, 12/e, p 315.)* In aortic regurgitation, much of the blood ejected during systole reenters the left ventricle during diastole. The ventricle dilates and the end-diastolic volume is increased. The left ventricular stroke volume has to be increased to handle the blood normally entering from the atrium in addition to the blood that returns from the aorta. The forward cardiac output is thus normal or decreased. The pulse pressure is widened because of the elevated systolic pressure (brought about by the increased stroke volume) and reduced diastolic pressure (as a consequence of backflow of blood through the incompetent aortic valve). The increased volume load on the heart causes ventricular hypertrophy.

83–85. The answers are 83-D, 84-C, 85-E. *(Berne, 3/e, pp 368–375.)* The action potential of the ventricular muscle is initiated when the membrane potential is depolarized to threshold. At threshold, sodium channels are activated, which increases the flow of sodium into the cell and causes the rapid upstroke of the action potential. Membrane depolarization causes inactivation of the sodium channels and is responsible for the small phase I repolarization (point C). Inactivation of sodium channels, however, does not cause the membrane to return to its resting potential. Instead the membrane remains depolarized, producing the plateau phase (phase 2) of the action potential. Phase 2 (point D) is associated with an increase in calcium conductance and a decrease in potassium conductance. The increase in calcium conductance is caused by the opening of calcium channels. The amount of calcium entering the cell during the plateau phase influences the strength of the heart beat. Norepinephrine increases contractility by increasing the flow of calcium into the cell. Various calcium blocking agents, such as nifedipine and verapamil, decrease contractility by diminishing the amount of calcium entering the ventricular cells. Repolarization (phase 3, point E) in ventricular muscle cells is caused by the opening of a calcium-activated potassium channel. The calcium flowing into the cell during the plateau is responsible for activating this channel.

86–87. The answers are 86–B, 87–E. *(West, 12/e, p 181.)* The ECG tracing represents the propagation of the cardiac action potentials through the heart. The P wave represents the electrical activity associated with atrial depolarization, the QRS wave represents the depolarization of the ventricular muscle, and the T wave represents the repolarization of the ventricular muscle. Depolarization of the His bundles and Purkinje fibers occurs during interval B, that is, in the isoelectric period of the ECG between the end of the P wave and the beginning of the QRS complex (the PR segment). This electrical activity is not represented on the normal ECG because it is too small. The aortic valve closes when the pressure in the ventricle drops below that in the aorta. Ventricular pressure begins to fall during period E, that is, when the ventricular muscle repolarizes.

88–90. The answers are 88–F, 89–C, 90–A. *(Berne, 3/e, pp 410–412.)* The left ventricular pressure-volume loop represents the changes in pressure and volume that occur during a cardiac cycle. The change in pressure and volume during diastole is represented by the curve G–A. The mitral valve opens at point G. As blood flows into the ventricle, its volume and pressure increase. Diastole ends when the ventricle begins to contract. Point A represents the end of diastole and the beginning of the isovolumic contraction phase. Point A is also the point at which the mitral valve closes and the first heart sound begins. The line A–B–C represents isovolumic contraction. During this phase of the cardiac cycle, pressure within the ventricle is increasing without any change in volume. Isovolumic contraction ends and ejection begins at point C. Point C is also the point at which the pressure in the ventricle exceeds the pressure in the aorta and the aortic valve opens. The curve C–D–E represents ejection. Ejection ends at point E when the pressure in the ventricle falls below that of the aorta. This is the point at which the second heart sound begins and the aortic valve closes. It is also the point at which isovolumic relaxation begins. Following the closure of the aortic valve, the ventricle begins to relax. The line E–F–G represents isovolumic relaxation. Point F occurs during isovolumic relaxation. During this phase of the cardiac cycle, pressure in the ventricle falls with no change in ventricular volume. Point G presents the end of isovolumic relaxation and the beginning of diastole. At this point, the pressure in the left atrium exceeds the pressure in the left ventricle and blood flows into the ventricle and a new cardiac cycle begins.

91–94. The answers are 91-B, 92-E, 93-F, 94-B. *(West, 12/e, pp 239–242.)* The graph accompanying the questions illustrates the development of pressure in the aorta and left atrium and ventricle during the cardiac cycle. A similar set of tracings would be obtained simultaneously from the pulmonary artery and right atrium and ventricle. The magnitude of the pressures attained during systole is lower on the right side. In addition, since pulmonary artery pressure is much lower than aortic pressure, the pulmonic valve opens sooner and right ventricular ejection begins before left ventricular ejection.

During diastole, when the atrioventricular valves are open and the ventricles are filling, atrial and ventricular pressures are identical. Atrial systole or contraction occurring at the end of diastole causes a transient increase in both atrial and ventricular pressures, which ends at point B when the mitral valve closes. Ventricular systole begins with the onset of isovolumetric ventricular contraction (point B). This initial part of systole lasts for 60 ms in the left ventricle and 15 ms in the right ventricle because the right ventricle has to develop less pressure to open the pulmonic valve. During this phase, which ends at point C, both the atrioventricular (mitral) and semilunar (aortic) valves are closed and no further change in ventricular volume occurs. The transient increase in atrial pressure occurring during this interval reflects the bulging of the mitral valve leaflets into the atrium as ventricular pressure rises. With the opening of the aortic valve (point C), ventricular ejection begins. During ventricular ejection, which lasts for 200 ms in the left ventricle and 270 ms in the right ventricle, aortic and left ventricular pressures are nearly identical. Atrial pressure declines initially as the ventricles move away from the atria, but then it gradually rises because of continued atrial filling. As the ventricles begin to relax, both ventricular pressure and aortic pressure fall. When left ventricular pressure falls below aortic pressure (point E), the aortic valve closes. This marks the beginning of isovolumetric ventricular relaxation, which lasts for 100 ms and during which no flow occurs because both the aortic and mitral valves are closed. When ventricular pressure falls below atrial pressure, the mitral valve opens (point F) and ventricular filling (diastole) begins. During the initial filling phase of diastole, both atrial and ventricular pressures decline and ventricular filling is rapid. This is followed by a longer slow filling phase during which atrial and ventricular pressures are the same and gradually rise. This slow filling phase is variable in length; its duration is reduced as heart rate increases.

95–98. The answers are 95-D, 96-E, 97-B, 98-A. *(Berne, 3/e, pp 408–409, 425–429, 436, 500–505.)* Starling's law of the heart states that increasing preload increases the force of contraction. The curves shown in the questions illustrate that relationship by plotting stroke volume as a function of end-diastolic volume (preload). If there is no other change, increasing the preload by increasing the blood volume will result in an increase in stroke volume (point C to point D). The acidosis resulting from myocardial ischemia would reduce contractility and cause a shift in the Starling curve (point C to point E). Pericardial effusion, on the other hand, would prevent normal filling of the heart and therefore cause a shift along the same Starling curve (point C to point B). A reduction in afterload would be indistinguishable from an increase in contractility, causing a shift in the Starling curve from point C to point A. It can therefore be seen that changes in preload cause shifts along the Starling curve, whereas changes in contractility or afterload cause a shift in the Starling curve.

99–100. The answers are 99-D, 100-C. *(Guyton, 8/e, pp 197, 202.)* Heart rate and blood pressure are regulated by the interaction of the sympathetic and parasympathetic divisions of the autonomic nervous system and medullary centers. Increases in heart rate are generally accompanied by increases in blood pressure. The net effect of both actions is to increase blood flow and improve perfusion.

An increase in intracranial pressure, which compresses cerebral vessels, results in decreased cerebral blood flow. The decrease in flow stimulates both the vasomotor and cardioinhibitory centers, elevating blood pressure and decreasing heart rate.

In exercise, impulses from the cerebral cortex converging on medullary centers as well as direct cardiac sympathetic stimulation result in an increase in blood pressure and tachycardia. During aerobic exercise, total peripheral resistance falls. In extreme cases, this can actually cause a decrease in blood pressure.

In hypoxia, chemoreceptor input into the vasomotor center produces an acceleration of heart rate and an increase in blood pressure. The net effect is improved oxygen delivery to peripheral areas.

Syncope, or fainting, is usually caused by an increase in vagal tone accompanied by a decrease in vasomotor activity. In some cases, the drop in blood pressure stimulates the baroreceptor reflex of the carotid sinus, which causes an increase in heart rate.

Vascular Physiology

DIRECTIONS: Each question below contains five suggested responses. Select the **one best** response to each question.

101. Immediate compensatory reactions to hemorrhagic shock include

(A) decreased peripheral resistance
(B) constriction of the vessels of the brain and heart
(C) reduced levels of circulating catecholamines
(D) excessive loss of Na^+ in the urine
(E) none of the above

102. The constriction of a blood vessel to one-half of its resting diameter would increase its resistance to blood flow by a factor of

(A) 2
(B) 4
(C) 8
(D) 12
(E) 16

103. Which one of the following best describes the function of AV anastomoses in the skin?

(A) Dilation of these vessels decreases blood flow to the skin
(B) Dilation of these vessels decreases heat loss
(C) These vessels are constricted by sympathetic stimulation
(D) These vessels are dilated by parasympathetic stimulation
(E) Constriction of these vessels increases blood flow to the subpapillary venous plexus.

104. Which one of the following would cause a reduction in arterial pulse pressure?

(A) A decrease in arterial compliance
(B) A decrease in venous compliance
(C) A decrease in blood volume
(D) An increase in central venous pressure
(E) An increase in myocardial contractility

105. When a person moves from the supine position to the standing position, there is an increase in

(A) central venous pressure
(B) preload
(C) heart rate
(D) the frequency of depolarization in the carotid sinus nerve
(E) stroke volume

106. Filtration of fluid out of the capillaries will be increased by

(A) an increase in precapillary resistance
(B) a decrease in postcapillary resistance
(C) an increase in plasma colloid osmotic pressure
(D) a decrease in mean blood pressure
(E) an increase in ventricular end-diastolic pressure

107. Central venous pressure is increased by

(A) decreasing blood volume
(B) increasing venous compliance
(C) increasing total peripheral resistance
(D) decreasing heart rate
(E) decreasing plasma aldosterone concentration

108. The increase in skeletal muscle blood flow that occurs during vigorous aerobic exercise

(A) causes an increase in total peripheral resistance
(B) causes an increase in blood pressure
(C) is primarily due to parasympathetic stimulation of skeletal muscle resistance vessels
(D) is primarily due to sympathetic stimulation of blood vessels
(E) is primarily the result of the accumulation of vasoactive metabolites

109. Blood flow through an organ would be increased by decreasing

(A) the diameter of the arterial vessels
(B) the number of open arterial vessels
(C) arterial pressure
(D) the diameter of the venous vessels
(E) hematocrit

110. Which one of the following is greater in pulmonary arterial vessels than in systemic arterial vessels?

(A) Blood flow
(B) Blood pressure
(C) Resistance
(D) Constriction induced by hypoxia
(E) Constriction induced by sympathetic stimulation

111. A reduction in carotid sinus pressure would cause a decrease in

(A) heart rate
(B) myocardial contractility
(C) total peripheral resistance
(D) venous capacitance
(E) cardiac output

112. Which one of the following organs has the highest arteriovenous O_2 difference under normal resting conditions?

(A) Brain
(B) Heart
(C) Skeletal muscle
(D) Kidney
(E) Stomach

113. The percentage of the total cardiac output distributed to any single organ is most dependent on

(A) the contractile state of the heart
(B) the magnitude of mean blood pressure
(C) the magnitude of diastolic pressure
(D) the ratio of an organ's vascular resistance to total peripheral resistance (TPR)
(E) the magnitude of cardiac output

114. At which of the following sites does the blood flow lose the greatest amount of energy?

(A) Mitral valve
(B) Large arteries
(C) Arterioles
(D) Capillaries
(E) Venules

115. Which of the following would most likely cause a reduction in pulse pressure?

(A) Arteriovenous fistula
(B) Aortic regurgitation
(C) Severe dehydration
(D) Hypertension
(E) Atherosclerosis

116. Which one of the following conditions would most likely cause the aortic and ventricular pressure waves diagrammed below?

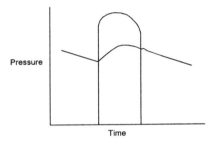

(A) Aortic regurgitation
(B) Aortic stenosis
(C) Increased ventricular contractility
(D) Mitral stenosis
(E) Atherosclerosis

117. Venous pressure in the dural sinuses normally falls within which of the following ranges?

(A) Subatmospheric
(B) 0 to 5 mmHg
(C) 5 to 10 mmHg
(D) 10 to 20 mmHg
(E) Greater than 20 mmHg

118. Which of the following statements regarding the flow of blood through the vascular bed pictured below (the numbers are the radii) is true?

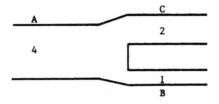

(A) The resistance of vessel C is two times the resistance of vessel A
(B) The resistance of vessel C is eight times the resistance of vessel A
(C) The flow through vessel C is twice the flow through vessel B
(D) The flow through vessel C is four times the flow through vessel B
(E) None of the above

119. Which one of the following characteristics is most similar in the systemic and pulmonary circulations?

(A) Stroke work
(B) Preload
(C) Afterload
(D) Peak systolic pressure
(E) Blood volume

120. Which of the following statements regarding closure of the ductus arteriosus is true?

(A) It reduces the flow of blood from the placenta to the vena cava
(B) It is stimulated by an increase in arterial P_{O_2}
(C) It interrupts a physiologic left-to-right shunt in the fetal circulation
(D) It is stimulated by prostacyclin
(E) None of the above

121. The hemoglobin-oxygen saturation of blood entering the right ventricle is approximately

(A) 95 percent
(B) 85 percent
(C) 75 percent
(D) 55 percent
(E) 35 percent

122. Occlusion of both carotid arteries between the heart and the carotid sinuses would be expected to produce

(A) increased blood pressure as measured in the femoral artery
(B) decreased heart rate
(C) increased activity in the afferent nerves from the carotid sinuses
(D) decreased activity of the vasomotor center
(E) decreased venous tone

123. Which of the following changes in perfusion of an organ system is an example of autoregulation?

(A) The decrease in renal blood flow during hemorrhage
(B) The decrease in blood flow to the skin during exposure to a cold environment
(C) The increase in coronary perfusion during exercise
(D) The increase in cerebral blood flow during hypercapnia
(E) None of the above

124. The venous system can act as a reservoir for peripheral blood chiefly because of the

(A) low compliance of the venous wall
(B) absence of smooth muscle fibers in the venous wall
(C) superficial location of the veins
(D) large volume capacity of the venous system
(E) low oxygen saturation in the venous system

125. The greatest percentage of blood volume is found in the

(A) heart
(B) aorta
(C) distributing arteries and arterioles
(D) capillaries
(E) venules and veins

126. Which of the following statements regarding activation of plasminogen is true?

(A) It follows a sequence of reactions involving serine proteases
(B) It occurs in blood but not in urine
(C) It is increased by vasodilatation
(D) It is inhibited by fibrin degradation products
(E) None of the above

127. *Diapedesis* is a term related to

(A) clotting
(B) pavementing
(C) cardiac arrest
(D) migration of neutrophils
(E) sickle cell anemia

128. Citrate is a useful anticoagulant because of its ability to

(A) buffer basic groups of coagulation factors
(B) bind factor XII
(C) bind vitamin K
(D) chelate calcium
(E) be slowly metabolized

129. Bleeding time is determined by nicking the skin superficially with a scalpel blade and measuring the time required for hemostasis. It will be markedly abnormal (prolonged) in a person who

(A) lacks factor VIII
(B) cannot absorb vitamin K
(C) has liver disease
(D) takes large quantities of aspirin
(E) takes coumarin derivatives

130. Lymph capillaries differ from systemic blood capillaries in that they

(A) are less permeable
(B) are not lined by endothelium
(C) lack valves
(D) are absent in the central nervous system
(E) collapse when interstitial pressure increases

131. Correct statements about the increase in pulmonary blood flow during vigorous exercise include which of the following?

(A) The percentage of increase in flow is greater in the bases of the lungs than in the apices
(B) The increase in flow is caused by a greater-than-fivefold increase in pulmonary arterial pressure
(C) The increase in pulmonary blood flow is less than the increase in systemic blood flow
(D) The increase in pulmonary blood flow is accommodated by dilation of pulmonary arterioles and capillaries
(E) The increase in pulmonary blood flow is caused by sympathetic nerve stimulation of the pulmonary vasculature

132. Pulmonary lymph flow exceeds that in other tissues because

(A) pulmonary capillary pressure is higher than systemic capillary pressure
(B) pulmonary endothelial cells contain a large number of fenestrations
(C) alveolar epithelial cells secrete a fluid that is added to the lymph formed from the blood plasma
(D) pulmonary interstitial fluids contain more plasma proteins than the interstitial fluid in other tissues
(E) pulmonary capillaries have a lower oncotic pressure than systemic capillaries

133. Cerebral blood flow may be increased by increasing

(A) ventilation
(B) central venous pressure
(C) pH
(D) arterial blood pressure
(E) carbon dioxide tension

134. At birth, changes that occur in the fetal circulation include

(A) increased systemic arterial pressure
(B) increased pulmonary vascular resistance
(C) increased pulmonary arterial pressure
(D) decreased left atrial pressure
(E) decreased pulmonary blood flow

135. Turbulence is more likely to occur in a blood vessel if

(A) the velocity of blood within the vessel increases
(B) the viscosity of blood within the vessel increases
(C) the diameter of the vessel decreases
(D) the density of the blood decreases
(E) the length of the vessel increases

136. Systemic arteriolar constriction may result from an increase in the local concentration of

(A) nitric oxide
(B) angiotensin II
(C) atrial natriuretic peptide
(D) beta agonists
(E) hydrogen ion

137. Increasing cytoplasmic calcium concentration within platelets stimulates

(A) activation of phospholipase C
(B) activation of phospholipase A_2
(C) elevation of cyclic-AMP concentration
(D) formation of protein kinase C
(E) inhibition of prostaglandin synthesis

DIRECTIONS: Each numbered question or incomplete statement below is NEGATIVELY phrased. Select the **one best** lettered response.

138. In which of the following organs will the rate of blood flow change the LEAST during exercise?

(A) Skin
(B) Brain
(C) Intestine
(D) Heart
(E) Kidney

139. In general, the percentage of the cardiac output flowing to a particular organ is related to the metabolic activity of that organ in comparison with the other organs of the body. This relationship is true for all the following EXCEPT the

(A) brain
(B) heart
(C) skeletal musculature
(D) intestine
(E) kidney

140. Cerebral blood flow is influenced by all the following EXCEPT

(A) viscosity of the blood
(B) P_{O_2} of the arterial blood
(C) cerebrospinal fluid pressure
(D) pH of the interstitial fluid of the brain
(E) vasomotor reflexes

141. Lymph flow is increased by all the following EXCEPT

(A) elevated capillary pressure
(B) elevated plasma protein concentration
(C) elevated interstitial fluid protein concentration
(D) bradykinin
(E) exercise

142. Hemorrhage generates all the following compensatory reactions EXCEPT

(A) arterial vasoconstriction
(B) venous vasoconstriction
(C) increased secretion of catecholamines
(D) bradycardia
(E) hemodilution

143. All the following substances involved in platelet activation are derived from the platelets EXCEPT

(A) thrombin
(B) thromboxane A_2
(C) adenosine diphosphate
(D) prostaglandin H_2 (PGH_2)
(E) calcium

144. Following the loss of blood, the LEAST likely event is an increase in

(A) heart rate
(B) sympathetic activity
(C) stroke volume
(D) total peripheral resistance
(E) ejection fraction

145. As a result of reduced stretch of the carotid baroreceptors, all the following would increase EXCEPT

(A) cardiac output
(B) heart rate
(C) total peripheral resistance (TPR)
(D) sympathetic nerve activity
(E) parasympathetic nerve activity

146. Which one of the following would NOT contribute to local hemostasis?

(A) Exposure of platelets to collagen
(B) The conversion of prothrombin to thrombin
(C) The conversion of plasminogen to plasmin
(D) The conversion of fibrinogen to fibrin
(E) The release of thromboxane A_2

DIRECTIONS: The group of questions below consists of lettered headings following by a set of numbered items. For each numbered item select the **one** lettered heading with which it is **most** closely associated. Each lettered heading may be used **once, more than once, or not at all**.

Questions 147–148

Use the diagram below to match each shift in cardiac output and central venous pressure with the most likely cause.

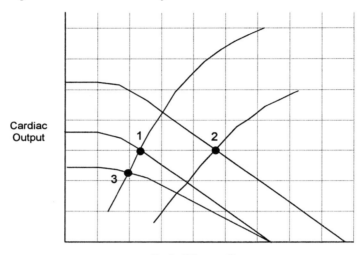

Central Venous Pressure

(A) An increase in contractility
(B) An increase in blood volume
(C) An increase in venous compliance
(D) An increase in total peripheral resistance
(E) An increase in heart rate

147. A shift in cardiac output and central venous pressure from point 1 to point 2

148. A shift in cardiac output and central venous pressure from point 1 to point 3

Vascular Physiology
Answers

101. The answer is E. *(Berne, 3/e, pp 537–540.)* Loss of blood volume leads to generalized vasoconstriction, with the exception of the vessels of the brain and heart. Peripheral resistance increases, although in irreversible shock it may fall. Sympathetic discharge as well as increased adrenal medullary secretion contribute to the increase in circulating catecholamines. Elevated levels of circulating catecholamines probably contribute relatively little to the generalized vasoconstriction but may lead to stimulation of the reticular formation. Sodium retention is marked in hemorrhagic shock, a phenomenon that favors reexpansion of blood volume.

102. The answer is E. *(Berne, 3/e, pp 240–243.)* According to Poiseuille's law, resistance is inversely proportional to the fourth power of the radius ($R \propto \frac{1}{r^4}$). Therefore, if the radius of a blood vessel is decreased by a factor of 2, the resistance to blood flow would increase by a factor of 2^4, or by 16 times.

103. The answer is C. *(Berne, 3/e, p 517.)* The AV anastomoses in the skin are direct connections between the arterial and venous vessels. The diameter of these vessels appears to be controlled almost exclusively by the sympathetic nervous system. They are not innervated by parasympathetic nerves. Dilation of these vessels causes a pronounced decrease in skin vascular resistance and, therefore, an increase in blood flow. Since they directly connect the arterial and venous vessels, dilation of the AV anastomoses increases blood flow to the subpapillary venous plexus.

104. The answer is C. *(Berne, 3/e, pp 460–462.)* The two major factors that influence pulse pressure are stroke volume and arterial compliance. Decreasing stroke volume reduces pulse pressure, whereas decreasing arterial compliance increases pulse pressure. A decrease in venous compliance would cause an increase in central venous pressure, which would tend to increase stroke volume. An increase in myocardial contractility would also tend to increase stroke volume and, therefore, pulse pressure. A reduction in blood volume leads to a decrease in stroke volume and, therefore, a decrease in pulse pressure.

105. The answer is C. *(Berne, 3/e, pp 505–507.)* As one moves from the supine position to the standing position, gravitational forces cause pooling of blood in the veins of the dependent portions of the body. This results in a decrease in central venous pressure and a decrease in preload, which would cause stroke volume to decrease. The decrease in stroke volume would result in a decrease in cardiac output and, therefore, blood pressure. The frequency of depolarization in the carotid sinus nerve decreases when blood pressure is reduced. A baroreceptor reflex would be initiated to compensate for the reduction in blood pressure. Part of the reflex response would be an increase in heart rate.

106. The answer is E. *(Guyton, 8/e, pp 172–175, 250.)* Fluid filtration out of the capillaries is increased by physiologic changes that cause either an increase in capillary hydrostatic pressure or a decrease in colloid osmotic pressure. Increasing precapillary resistance or decreasing postcapillary resistance would cause a reduction in capillary hydrostatic pressure. A decrease in mean blood pressure would also cause hydrostatic pressure in the capillaries to decrease. An increase in ventricular end-diastolic pressure would cause venous pressure to increase, which in turn would require capillary hydrostatic pressure to increase. Increasing end-diastolic pressure of the right ventricle causes an increase in fluid filtration from systemic capillaries. Increasing the end-diastolic pressure of the left ventricle increases fluid filtration from the pulmonary capillaries. Edema results from an increased fluid filtration in these areas.

107. The answer is D. *(Berne, 3/e, pp 494–504.)* Central venous pressure is the hydrostatic pressure in the great veins at their entrance to the right atrium. Increasing venous compliance would decrease pressure in the venous vessels and therefore would decrease central venous pressure. Decreasing blood volume would have the same effect. Reducing the plasma concentration of aldosterone would result in a decrease in blood volume. Increasing total peripheral resistance would tend to shift volume from the venous side of the circulation to the arterial side, resulting in a decrease in venous pressure. Increasing cardiac output tends to lower central venous pressure, whereas lowering cardiac output tends to increase central venous pressure. A reduction in heart rate would tend to lower cardiac output and therefore increase central venous pressure.

108. The answer is E. *(Berne, 3/e, pp 520–521, 532–535.)* During vigorous aerobic exercise there is a pronounced decrease in vascular resistance in skeletal muscle, which lowers total peripheral resistance. If it were not for the increase in cardiac output that occurs with this kind of exercise, blood pressure would decrease. The primary factor that contributes to the increase in blood flow to exercising skeletal muscles is the local accumulation of vasoactive metabolites. Stimulation of sympathetic nerve fibers that innervate blood vessels within exercising skeletal muscle would tend to increase vascular resistance and decrease flow. Local metabolites overpower the effects of sympathetic stimulation so that flow can increase despite high levels of sympathetic activity.

109. The answer is E. *(Berne, 3/e, pp 443–451.)* Blood flow through an organ is increased by either increasing the perfusion pressure across the organ or by decreasing the vascular resistance. A decrease in the arterial pressure would decrease the perfusion pressure. Decreasing the diameter of the arterial or venous vessels or decreasing the number of open arterial vessels would contribute to increasing vascular resistance. If the hematocrit is decreased, the viscosity of the blood is decreased, resulting in a decrease in resistance and, therefore, an increase in blood flow through an organ.

110. The answer is D. *(Berne, 3/e, pp 578–579.)* Since the pulmonary arterial vessels and the systemic arterial vessels are connected in series, blood flow through these segments is the same. Mean blood pressure in the systemic and pulmonary circulations equals the product of blood flow and resistance (MBP = CO • PR, where MBP = the mean pressure in the pulmonary or systemic circulation, CO = the output of the left or right ventricles, and PR = the total resistance of the systemic or pulmonary vascular systems). Since blood flow is the same in the systemic and pulmonary circulations and pulmonary vascular resistance is much lower than systemic vascular resistance, the mean blood pressure is much lower in the pulmonary arterial vessels. The systemic arterial vessels are much more responsive to sympathetic stimulation. In most cases, hypoxia causes dilation of the systemic arterial vessels and constriction of the pulmonary arterial vessels.

111. The answer is D. *(Berne, 3/e, pp 486–489, 538–539.)* A reduction in carotid sinus pressure due to a decrease in mean blood pressure would elicit a baroreceptor reflex tending to restore blood pressure to normal. The reflex response includes an increase in sympathetic nervous system activity, which would cause an increase in heart rate and myocardial contractility, both of which would tend to increase cardiac output. Sympathetic stimulation would also cause constriction of both the arterioles and venous vessels. Arteriolar constriction would cause an increase in total peripheral resistance. Sympathetic stimulation of the venous vessels would cause a decrease in venous capacitance.

112. The answer is B. *(Berne, 3/e, pp 510–525, 596.)* The overall arteriovenous O_2 difference is determined by the oxygen consumption of a tissue and its blood flow. Because of the high rate of metabolism in the heart compared with its blood flow, it has the highest arteriovenous O_2 difference of any major organ of the body under normal conditions. The heart can extract a large amount of oxygen because of its high capillary density. Blood flow to the kidney and skin is far in excess of their metabolic needs, so little oxygen is removed from the blood as it passes through these organs; therefore, their arteriovenous O_2 differences are rather small. Under normal conditions, the arteriovenous O_2 difference in skeletal muscle is quite low. However, this value can increase substantially during vigorous exercise.

113. The answer is D. *(Berne, 3/e, pp 444–446.)* The major organs of the body are supplied by arterial vessels arranged in parallel. The distribution of blood flow through a parallel network of vessels is determined by the relative resistance of each parallel pathway. The ratio of that resistance to the total resistance will determine the percentage of flow going through each of the parallel networks. The other factors mentioned will influence the magnitude of the cardiac output, which is the total amount of blood flowing through the entire system. However, none of these factors have any direct effect on the way blood flow is distributed to the organs of the body.

114. The answer is C. *(Berne, 3/e, pp 443–444.)* The energy imparted to the blood by ventricular systole is dissipated as the blood flows through the circulation. The greatest energy loss occurs where the resistance to blood flow is greatest. This would also be the site of the greatest pressure change. The arteriolar vessels produce the largest resistance to blood, and thus the greatest energy loss and pressure drop occur as the blood passes through them. Normal mitral valves offer almost no resistance to flow and thus there is almost no difference between ventricular pressure and atrial pressure during diastole. This explains why left atrial pressure, as evaluated by pulmonary capillary wedge pressure, can be used as an index of left ventricular end-diastolic pressure in patients with normal mitral valves. Under normal conditions, venous vessels contribute very little to vascular resistance.

115. The answer is C. *(Berne, 3/e, pp 553–562.)* Pulse pressure in the arterial system is primarily influenced by the stroke volume and the compliance of the arterial system. Aortic regurgitation and arteriovenous fistulas both increase stroke volume and therefore pulse pressure. Hypertension reduces arterial compliance indirectly. When mean blood pressure rises, the volume of the blood in the arterial system increases, and as a result the aorta is stretched. Stretching the aortic wall decreases its compliance. The plaque that builds up on the arterial wall during the development of atherosclerosis directly causes a reduction in arterial compliance. The reduction in compliance associated with hypertension and atherosclerosis leads to an increase in pulse pressure. Severe dehydration reduces blood volume, leading to a decrease in preload and, therefore, a reduction in stroke volume. The reduction in stroke volume causes a reduction in pulse pressure.

116. The answer is B. *(Guyton, 8/e, p 257.)* The ventricular pressure illustrated in the diagram is much higher than the aortic pressure. The pressure difference between the left ventricle and aorta during ejection results from a large resistance across the aortic valve as would occur with aortic stenosis. Under normal conditions, the aortic valve offers almost no resistance to flow and therefore there would be virtually no pressure gradient between the left ventricle and the aorta.

117. The answer is A. *(Guyton, 8/e, pp 681–683.)* Normal right atrial pressure is approximately 5 mmHg. Because of hydrostatic pressure, in the standing position venous pressure in the legs is greater than central venous pressure, whereas pressure in the head and neck is less. In the neck, normal veins collapse when a person is in an upright position; intracranially, the dural sinuses, having more rigid walls, are unable to collapse and sinus pressure may drop below 0 mmHg. During an intracranial operation upon a patient in a sitting position, the resultant negative pressure presents a danger that atmospheric air may be drawn into an exposed sinus and thus cause an air embolus.

118. The answer is E. *(Berne, 3/e, pp 441–447.)* Resistance of a blood vessel is proportional to $1/(radius)^4$. Since the radius of C is one-half the radius of A, it has 16 times the resistance of A. The flow through two vessels in parallel is proportional to 1/resistance. Since vessel C is twice the radius of B, it has $\frac{1}{16}$ the resistance and thus 16 times the flow.

119. The answer is B. *(West, 12/e, pp 112, 529–532.)* The right and left ventricles are in series with one another so that the entire cardiac output (except for a small anatomic shunt) passes through both circulations. Since the two ventricles beat at the same rate, their stroke volumes are the same. However, the resistance of the pulmonary vasculature is much smaller than that of the systemic circulation; thus the afterload and stroke work are greater on the left side than on the right side. Because the same cardiac output is ejected into a higher resistance, peak systolic pressure is higher on the left side than on the right side. Only about 10 percent of the blood volume is within the pulmonary circulation at any one time. About two-thirds of the blood volume is stored within the systemic veins and venules. Although the left and right preloads are not identical, they are very similar.

120. The answer is B. *(Guyton, 8/e, pp 259–261.)* The ductus arteriosus connects the aorta and pulmonary artery and functions as a physiologic right-to-left shunt during fetal life because the lungs are collapsed and pulmonary vascular resistance is higher than systemic resistance. At birth, the lungs expand and pulmonary vascular resistance and pulmonary artery pressure fall drastically, while systemic vascular resistance and pressure rise owing to removal of the low-resistance placental circulation. Blood flow through the ductus is then reversed. Within a few hours the elevated P_{O_2} in the aortic blood passing through the ductus causes it to constrict and finally to close completely within a few weeks. When the ductus arteriosus fails to close spontaneously, surgical ligation may be necessary. Since the patency of the ductus is maintained in part by prostacyclin, inhibitors of prostaglandin synthesis such as indomethacin have been used to induce ductus closure and avoid surgery.

121. The answer is C. *(Berne, 3/e, pp 590–592.)* The hemoglobin-oxygen dissociation curve is sigmoidal. Normally P_{O_2} and hemoglobin saturation lie at the top of the curve so that hemoglobin saturation varies over a narrow range. Under physiologic conditions, the P_{O_2} of arterial blood is 100 mmHg and hemoglobin is approximately 98 percent saturated with oxygen. Some venous blood bypasses the lungs and prevents saturation from reaching 100 percent. Blood entering the right ventricle represents venous blood where P_{O_2} is at its lowest (40 mmHg) and hemoglobin saturation reaches its minimum of 75 percent.

122. The answer is A. *(Berne, 3/e, pp 420–421, 486–489.)* The carotid sinuses contain baroreceptors that respond to distention by discharging at an increased rate when arterial pressure rises. Impulses from these receptors inhibit the vasomotor center in the brainstem and cause vasodilation. They also excite the cardioinhibitory center and cause bradycardia. Occlusion of the carotid arteries between the heart and the carotid sinuses would decrease the pressure in the sinus and remove the inhibitory influences on the brainstem, which in turn would result in tachycardia and vasoconstriction with increased arterial pressure.

123. The answer is E. *(Berne, 3/e, p 101.)* Autoregulation is the maintenance of a constant blood flow in the presence of a change in arterial pressure. Two mechanisms have been used to explain autoregulation, the myogenic and metabolic theories. The myogenic theory proposes that an increase (or decrease) in perfusion pressure causes a contraction (or relaxation) of the arteriolar smooth muscle, thus reducing (or increasing) blood flow toward normal. The metabolic theory proposes that blood flow is adjusted to keep the concentration of metabolic by-products at a constant level. The changes in blood flow in response to overall homeostasis (e.g., the regulation of temperature or blood pressure during a hemorrhage) or specific tissue needs (e.g., the dilation of coronary arteries when the energy requirements of the heart increase during exercise) are not classified as autoregulatory processes.

124. The answer is D. *(Berne, 3/e, pp 495–497, 505–507.)* The vessels of the venous system contain a thinner smooth muscle coat than their arterial and arteriolar counterparts but are still capable of significant contraction. The venous system has a large volume capacity. Thus, the level of tone within the system is important in the adjustment of blood volume in response to exercise and the gravitational effects of postural change.

125. The answer is E. *(Berne 3/e, pp 330–332.)* The total circulating blood volume is approximately 70 mL/kg; about two-thirds is found in the systemic veins and venules. A significant volume of blood (15 percent) is found in the pulmonary circulation. Smaller quantities are found in the heart (5 percent), the arterial system (11 percent), and the capillaries (5 percent). The large volume of blood found on the venous side of the circulation is used to adjust circulating blood volume. For example, during hemorrhage, contraction of the veins and venules of the skin increases the amount of blood available for perfusion of the heart and brain.

126. The answer is C. *(West, 12/e, pp 397–398.)* Activation of plasminogen to plasmin, a serine protease that functions as the major fibrinolytic enzyme, occurs in both blood and urine by the action of different proteases. Vascular plasminogen activator is released from endothelial cells in response to stress, exercise, or vasodilatation and catalyzes the hydrolysis of plasminogen to plasmin while both are bound to a fibrin surface. It is rapidly cleared from the blood by the liver and has a half-life of only 15 min. Urokinase, the urinary plasminogen activator, catalyzes the cleavage in solution, thereby promoting fibrinolysis within renal tubules and preventing tubular occlusion. Cleavage of plasminogen to plasmin involves cleavage of a single arginine-valine bond. Fibrin degradation products released following fibrinolysis by plasmin inhibit hemostasis by interfering with the binding of fibrinogen to platelets.

127. The answer is D. *(Berne, 3/e, pp 330–332.)* Diapedesis is the process by which neutrophils pass through the endothelial layer and basement membrane of capillaries into surrounding tissue. Penetration of the vessel wall is preceded by margination and attachment of neutrophils to the capillary wall. This margination and migration occurs in response to chemotactic factors elaborated by bacteria or the immune system.

128. The answer is D. *(Guyton, 3/e, p 395.)* The citrate ion has three anionic carboxylate groups that avidly chelate calcium and reduce the concentration of free calcium in blood. Because free calcium (Ca^{2+}) is required for multiple steps in both coagulation pathways, citrate is a useful anticoagulant in vitro. The citrate ion is rapidly metabolized; thus blood anticoagulated with citrate can be infused into the body without untoward effects. Oxalate, another calcium-chelating anticoagulant, is toxic to cells.

129. The answer is D. *(West, 12/e, pp 385–389.)* Hemostasis following blood vessel injury depends on (1) vascular spasm, (2) formation of a platelet plug, and (3) clot formation. When injury to a vessel produces only a small defect, the platelet plug itself can cause hemostasis. This is the basis for the bleeding time that is employed clinically to distinguish hemostatic abnormalities caused by platelet abnormalities from those caused by coagulation defects. Aspirin diminishes platelet aggregation by inhibiting cyclooxygenase, an enzyme required for generation of thromboxanes, which promote platelet aggregation. All the other situations described in the question are associated with coagulation deficiency. Persons thus affected would have a normal bleeding time but would present clinically with delayed posttraumatic bleeding caused by their inability to form an effective clot to reinforce the platelet plug.

130. The answer is D. *(West, 12/e, pp 131–133.)* Nearly all tissues of the body have a lymphatic circulation, one exception being the central nervous system. The lymphatic channels (or capillaries), which ultimately drain into the venous circulation, are lined by endothelial cells. These cells are attached to surrounding tissues by anchoring filaments and have large gaps between them to permit the free movement of macromolecules and particulate matter such as bacteria. The endothelial gaps are covered by overlapping, loosely adherent cell processes that act as valves to prevent the backflow of fluid once it enters the lumen. Valves, as well, exist within the channels every few millimeters to promote unidirectional flow.

131. The answer is D. *(Berne, 3/e, pp 582–584. Guyton, 8/e, pp 415–418.)* The pulmonary circulation is a low-pressure system compared with the systemic circulation. Because of this low pressure and the hydrostatic pressure gradient from the top, or apex, of the lung to the bottom, or base, of the lung, the apex of the lung is not as well perfused as the base of the lung. During vigorous exercise there is a large (up to sixfold) increase in cardiac output. The increased flow through the systemic circulation is equal to the increase in flow through the pulmonary circulation. Total lung flow increases and flow at the base of the lung is still greater than flow at the apex. However, the flow at the apex, since it was originally low, may increase by up to 800 percent, whereas flow in the base of the lung only increases by up to about 300 percent. The pulmonary vessels are very compliant. The increased flow causes recruitment of previously closed capillaries and dilation of pulmonary arterioles and capillaries. Because of this, pulmonary artery pressure normally does not increase or increases by only a small amount, and it rarely increases more than twofold.

132. The answer is D. *(West, 12/e, pp 134–137.)* The rate of lymph flow is increased by factors that favor the flow of fluid from the capillaries to the interstitial spaces. Such factors include an elevation of capillary pressure, a decrease in plasma oncotic pressure, an increase in interstitial plasma proteins, and an increase in capillary permeability. The major factor involved in the increased formation of lymph within the lungs is the large leak of plasma proteins from the capillary to the interstitial fluid. The loss of plasma proteins from the capillaries occurs by diffusion through the spaces between capillary endothelial cells and not through endothelial cell fenestrations. The pressure within the pulmonary capillaries is lower than in systemic capillaries and so acts to reduce lymph formation. However, the negative intrapleural pressure acts to increase the pressure gradient across the capillary wall and so promotes lymph formation.

133. The answer is E. *(Berne, 3/e, pp 523–524.)* Cerebral blood flow is under local metabolic control. The increase in H^+, CO_2, and K^+ that accompanies neural activity causes an increase in cerebral blood flow. Hyperventilation causes a respiratory alkalosis, which, by decreasing brain H^+ concentration (increasing pH), decreases cerebral blood flow. Increasing central venous pressure decreases the perfusion pressure across the brain vasculature and thus impedes cerebral blood flow. The brain is protected from an increase in blood flow during hypertension by autoregulatory mechanisms.

134. The answer is A. *(Berne, 3/e, pp 527–529.)* At birth, two major events cause changes in the fetal circulation. First, loss of the placenta results in increased peripheral resistance and increased systemic arterial pressure. Second, expansion of the lungs allows marked pulmonary vasodilatation, which, by diminishing vascular resistance and promoting pulmonary blood flow, results in elevation of left atrial pressure.

135. The answer is A. *(West, 12/e, pp 143–144.)* The critical factors affecting the flow of incompressible fluids in pipes were described late in the nineteenth century by the English physicist Osborne Reynolds. He discovered that the point at which flow changes from laminar (smooth) to turbulent is a function of fluid density, viscosity, and velocity and of the diameter of the vessel, expressed in the relationship that became known as the Reynolds number (Re):

$$Re = \frac{density \times diameter \times velocity}{viscosity}$$

This relationship is equally valid for blood moving in the vessels of living organisms and for water moving in pipes. Increasing the length of the vessel may indirectly decrease the likelihood of turbulence by increasing vascular resistance and thus decreasing blood velocity.

136. The answer is B. *(Berne, 3/e, pp 540, 772–775. Guyton, 8/e, pp 191–193.)* Angiotensin II is a powerful vasoconstrictor that is formed when renin is released from the kidney in response to a fall in blood pressure or vascular volume. Renin converts angiotensinogen to angiotensin I. Angiotensin II is formed from angiotensin I by an angiotensin-converting enzyme localized within the vasculature of the lung. All the other listed substances cause vasodilation.

137. The answer is B. *(West, 12/e, pp 387–390.)* Activation of platelets at a site of injury is stimulated by thrombin and the exposed collagen on the blood vessel endothelium. The activation process involves a G-protein–mediated activation of phospholipase C, which hydrolyzes phosphatidylinositol-4,5-bisphosphate (PIP_2) to form diacylglycerol (DAG) and IP_3. The IP_3, in turn, releases Ca^{2+} from internal stores. The elevated cytoplasmic Ca^{2+} concentration then leads to the activation of phospholipase A_2, which causes the release of arachidonic acid from the platelet membrane. Protein kinase C is activated by DAG. Prostaglandins, particularly PGH_2, are formed from arachidonic acid by a reaction catalyzed by cyclooxygenase.

138. The answer is B. *(West, 12/e, pp 155–156, 303–304.)* During exercise, metabolism and cardiac output increase. Blood flow to the skin increases to aid in the dissipation of heat while blood flow to the heart increases to provide adequate oxygen and nutrients and to remove wastes. During exercise, systemic resistance falls because of the extensive vasodilation in the exercising muscles. Blood flow to the intestine and kidney decreases in order to maintain adequate blood pressure. Autoregulatory mechanisms within the cerebral circulation keep blood flow in the brain from changing.

139. The answer is E. *(Berne, 3/e, pp 736–739.)* The kidney receives approximately 20 percent of the cardiac output while consuming a much smaller portion of the body's oxygen consumption. The high renal blood flow is related to the kidney's role in regulating the composition of the extracellular fluid. The skin is another organ in which the relationship between percentage of blood flow and percentage of oxygen consumption does not hold. Blood flow to the skin is primarily related to its role in temperature regulation. Of course in all organs, if oxygen consumption increases, blood flow will increase.

140. The answer is E. *(Berne, 3/e, pp 523–524.)* Cerebral blood flow is held constant under varying conditions. It is influenced by intracranial pressure, arterial pressure, arterial P_{O_2} arterial and extracellular fluid pH, and blood viscosity. Vasomotor reflexes, mediated via the autonomic nervous system, have little part in controlling cerebral blood flow despite the fact that cerebral vessels are innervated by both sympathetic and parasympathetic fibers.

141. The answer is B. *(Guyton, 8/e, pp 180–183. West, 12/e, pp 134–136.)* Lymphatic flow is essential for maintenance of a low interstitial fluid protein concentration and for prevention of fluid accumulation in tissues. The rate of lymph flow is regulated by the net interstitial fluid pressure and the pumping activity of the lymphatic vessels. Interstitial fluid pressure is normally subatmospheric because the colloid osmotic pressure of plasma that draws fluid into blood capillaries exceeds the sum of the capillary perfusion pressure and interstitial fluid pressure. When this balance is altered, interstitial fluid pressure rises to a level above atmospheric pressure and lymph flow is increased drastically. Imbalances may be caused by (1) elevated capillary pressure (cardiac failure); (2) increased interstitial fluid protein concentration, such as would occur following an increase in capillary permeability induced by bradykinin; or (3) decreased plasma oncotic pressure. Compression of lymphatic channels during exercise also promotes lymph flow. Increased plasma protein concentration would increase plasma colloid osmotic pressure and cause retention of fluid within capillaries.

142. The answer is D. *(Berne, 3/e, pp 537–540.)* Reduction in blood volume by hemorrhage decreases venous return. The arterial baroreceptors are stretched to a lesser degree and sympathetic outflow is increased. There is reflex tachycardia and generalized vasoconstriction, except in the blood vessels of the brain and heart. Venoconstriction helps to maintain the filling pressure of the heart.

143. The answer is A. *(West, 12/e, pp 387–390.)* When platelets are exposed to a site of injury they are stimulated by thrombin and collagen. This stimulation activates (1) phospholipase C, which generates inositol triphosphate (IP_3), which in turn releases calcium from internal stores; and (2) phospholipase A_2, which generates arachidonic acid, which is then oxidized by cyclooxygenase to produce thromboxane A_2, and PGH_2. Both of these amplify platelet activation: thromboxane A_2 enhances the action of collagen and PGH_2

increases the activity of phospholipase C. Adenosine diphosphate (ADP) is released from dense core granules within platelets. It enhances platelet activation.

144. The answer is C. *(Berne, 3/e, pp 540–542.)* Following the loss of blood there is a reduction in preload, which results in a decrease in stroke volume. The direct consequence of the decrease in stroke volume is a reduction in cardiac output and secondarily a decrease in blood pressure. This reduction in blood pressure would be detected by the baroreceptors, leading to an increased activity of the sympathetic nervous system. Sympathetic stimulation would cause an increase in heart rate and total peripheral resistance. Sympathetic stimulation would also lead to an increase in myocardial contractility. An increase in ejection fraction could result from the increase in contractility and reduced afterload. All the reflex compensations described above help to return blood pressure to normal when stroke volume is reduced. Even if compensation were to correct the problem completely, stroke volume would at best be returned to the control value.

145. The answer is E. *(Berne, 3/e, pp 420, 538.)* The baroreceptor reflex decreases blood pressure when the mean arterial blood pressure suddenly rises and increases blood pressure when the mean arterial blood pressure suddenly falls. Stretch of the carotid sinus baroreceptors is reduced when there is a decrease in blood pressure, and therefore, the reflex responses to a reduced stretch of the carotid sinus baroreceptors all tend to increase blood pressure. These reflex responses include an increase in sympathetic nervous system activity and a decrease in activity of the vagal fibers that innervate the heart. Increasing sympathetic nervous system activity increases heart rate and contractility, which leads to increased cardiac output. Increased sympathetic nervous system activity also increases arteriolar tone, which increases total peripheral resistance and blood pressure. The reduced vagal nerve activity allows the heart rate to increase and thus contributes to the increase in cardiac output and blood pressure following a decreased stretch of the carotid sinus baroreceptors.

146. The answer is C. *(Berne, 3/e, pp 340–356.)* The activation of platelets and the formation of fibrin strands contribute to blood clotting and hemostasis. Exposure of platelets to collagen, thrombin, and thromboxane A_2 causes activation of the platelets. The conversion of fibrinogen to fibrin is essential for the production of fibrin strands to trap blood components in the forming clot. Plasmin is an enzyme that contributes to the lysis of blood clots. The injection of lytic drugs has become an important clinical tool in the prevention of myocardial infarction.

147–148. The answers are 147-B, 148-D. *(Berne, 3/e, pp 494–504.)* The graph illustrates two cardiac function curves (Starling curves) and three vascular function curves. Point 1 illustrates the normal situation and points 2 and 3 illustrate the situation after the cardiovascular system is altered. The shift in the vascular function curve from point 1 to point 2 could have resulted from either a decrease in venous compliance or an increase in blood volume. The shift in the cardiac function curve from point 1 to point 2 could have resulted from either a decrease in contractility or from an increase in afterload. However, afterload is the same at points 1 and 2. Afterload has not changed because blood pressure has not changed, and blood pressure has not changed because neither cardiac output nor total peripheral resistance has changed.

The change in the vascular function curve from point 1 to point 3 is caused by an increase in total peripheral resistance. When blood volume increases or decreases, there is a parallel shift in the vascular function curve. A downward shift (decrease in slope) of the vascular function curve represents an increase in total peripheral resistance. An upward shift in the vascular function curve represents a decrease in total peripheral resistance.

Gastrointestinal Physiology

DIRECTIONS: Each question below contains five suggested responses. Select the **one best** response to each question.

149. Chronic administration of antacids and maintenance of a gastric pH that is about 7 would cause gastrin levels to

(A) decrease
(B) increase
(C) decrease, then subsequently increase
(D) increase, then decrease
(E) remain unchanged

150. Which one of the following statements about small intestinal motility is correct?

(A) Contractile frequency is constant from duodenum to terminal ileum
(B) Peristalsis is the major contractile pattern during feeding
(C) Migrating motor complexes occur during the digestive period
(D) Vagotomy abolishes contractile activity during the digestive period
(E) Contractile activity is initiated in response to bowel wall distention

151. Which one of the following statements about gastric emptying is correct?

(A) Solids empty more rapidly than liquids
(B) Vagotomy accelerates the emptying of solids
(C) Undigestible food empties during the digestive period
(D) Acidification of the antrum decreases gastric emptying
(E) Vagotomy decreases accommodation of the proximal stomach

152. Vitamin B_{12} is absorbed primarily in the

(A) stomach
(B) duodenum
(C) jejunum
(D) ileum
(E) colon

153. The principal paracrine secretion involved in the inhibitory feedback regulation of gastric acid secretion is

(A) gastrin
(B) somatostatin
(C) histamine
(D) enterogastrone
(E) acetylcholine

154. Gastric acid secretion is increased by

(A) acidification of the antrum
(B) administration of H_2-receptor antagonists
(C) vagotomy
(D) duodenal ulcer disease
(E) gastric ulcer disease

155. Which one of the following is the putative inhibitory neurotransmitter responsible for relaxation of gastrointestinal smooth muscle?

(A) Dopamine
(B) Vasoactive intestinal peptide
(C) Somatostatin
(D) Substance P
(E) Acetylcholine

156. Which one of the following will inhibit gastric acid secretion?

(A) Gastrin
(B) Entero-oxyntin
(C) Somatostatin
(D) Acetylcholine
(E) Histamine

157. Cholera toxin causes diarrhea by inhibiting

(A) neutral NaCl absorption in the small intestine
(B) electrogenic Na absorption from the small intestine
(C) Na-glucose coupled absorption from the small intestine
(D) Na/H exchange in the small intestine
(E) electrogenic Na absorption from the colon

158. Which one of the following statements best describes water and electrolyte absorption in the GI tract?

(A) Most water and electrolytes come from ingested fluids
(B) The small intestine and colon have similar absorptive capacities
(C) Osmotic equilibration of chyme occurs in the stomach
(D) The majority of absorption occurs in the jejunum
(E) Water absorption is independent of Na^+ absorption

159. Hypokalemic, metabolic acidosis can occur with excess fluid loss from the

(A) stomach
(B) ileum
(C) colon
(D) pancreas
(E) liver

160. Which gastrointestinal motor activity is most affected by vagotomy?

(A) Secondary esophageal peristalsis
(B) Distention-induced intestinal segmentation
(C) Orad stomach accommodation
(D) Caudad stomach peristalsis
(E) Migrating motor complexes

161. The hormone involved in coordination of the migrating motor complex is

(A) gastrin
(B) motilin
(C) secretin
(D) cholecystokinin
(E) enterogastrone

162. The rate of gastric emptying increases with an increase in

(A) intragastric volume
(B) intraduodenal volume
(C) fat content of duodenum
(D) osmolality of duodenum
(E) acidity of duodenum

163. Which phase of secretion of acid will be most affected by a vagotomy?

(A) Basal
(B) Cephalic
(C) Gastric
(D) Interdigestive
(E) Intestinal

164. Which one of the following processes applies to the proximal stomach?

(A) Accommodation
(B) Peristalsis
(C) Retropulsion
(D) Segmentation
(E) Trituration

165. After secretion of trypsinogen into the duodenum, the enzyme is converted into its active form, trypsin, by

(A) enteropeptidase
(B) procarboxypeptidase
(C) pancreatic lipase
(D) previously secreted trypsin
(E) an alkaline pH

166. The major mechanism for absorption of sodium from the small intestine is

(A) nonelectrolytic cotransport
(B) cotransport with potassium
(C) electrogenic transport
(D) neutral NaCl absorption
(E) solvent drag

167. Pharmacologic blockade of histamine H_2 receptors in the gastric mucosa

(A) inhibits both gastrin-induced and vagally mediated secretion of acid
(B) inhibits gastrin-induced but not vagally mediated secretion of acid
(C) has no effect on either gastrin-induced or vagally mediated secretion of acid
(D) prevents activation of adenyl cyclase by gastrin
(E) causes an increase in potassium transport by gastric parietal (oxyntic) cells

168. Gallbladder contraction is controlled primarily by the hormone

(A) enterogastrone
(B) cholecystokinin-pancreozymin (CCK)
(C) insulin
(D) secretin
(E) glucagon

169. Mass movements (strong peristalsis) in the colon would be abolished by

(A) vagotomy
(B) extrinsic denervation
(C) distention of the colon
(D) destruction of Meissner's plexus
(E) destruction of Auerbach's plexus

170. Dietary fat, after being processed, is extruded from the mucosal cells of the gastrointestinal tract into the lymphatic ducts in the form of

(A) monoglycerides
(B) diglycerides
(C) triglycerides
(D) chylomicrons
(E) free fatty acids

171. Acute obstruction of the common bile duct produced experimentally will incur which of the following changes in plasma and urinary levels of bilirubin?

	Unconjugated bilirubin in plasma	Conjugated bilirubin in plasma	Conjugated bilirubin in urine
(A)	Increase	No change	Increase
(B)	No change	Increase	Increase
(C)	Decrease	Decrease	Decrease
(D)	Increase	Decrease	Increase
(E)	Decrease	No change	Increase

172. Gas within the colon is primarily derived from which one of the following sources?

(A) CO_2 liberated by the interaction of HCO_3^- and H^+
(B) Diffusion from the blood
(C) Fermentation of undigested oligosaccharides by bacteria
(D) Swallowed atmospheric air
(E) None of the above

173. Removal of the antrum is associated with

(A) a decrease in gastric compliance
(B) an increase in maximal output of acid
(C) an increase in basal output of acid
(D) an increase in the rate of gastric emptying of solids
(E) an increase in the serum gastrin level

174. Removal of the terminal ileum will result in

(A) a decrease in absorption of amino acids
(B) an increase in the water content of the feces
(C) an increase in the concentration of bile acid in the enterohepatic circulation
(D) a decrease in the fat content of the feces
(E) an increase in the absorption of iron

175. Vitamins synthesized by intestinal bacteria and absorbed in significant quantities include

(A) vitamin B_6
(B) vitamin K
(C) thiamine
(D) riboflavin
(E) folic acid

176. Secretion of acid by the gastric mucosa is correctly described by which one of the following statements?

(A) It is carried out by chief cells
(B) It is inhibited by acetylcholine
(C) It is inhibited by antihistamines taken by allergy patients
(D) It involves active transport of H^+
(E) It involves release of HCl from zymogen granules

177. Which one of the following statements about the colon is correct?

(A) Absorption of Na^+ in the colon is under hormonal (aldosterone) control
(B) Bile acids enhance absorption of water from the colon
(C) Net absorption of HCO_3^- occurs in the colon
(D) Net absorption of K^+ occurs in the colon
(E) The luminal potential in the colon is positive

178. Contraction of the gallbladder is correctly described by which one of the following statements?

(A) It is inhibited by a fat-rich meal
(B) It is inhibited by the presence of amino acids in the duodenum
(C) It is stimulated by atropine
(D) It occurs in response to cholecystokinin
(E) It occurs simultaneously with the contraction of the sphincter of Oddi

179. Acidification of the duodenum will

(A) decrease pancreatic secretion of bicarbonate
(B) increase secretion of gastric acid
(C) decrease gastric emptying
(D) increase contraction of the gallbladder
(E) increase contraction of the sphincter of Oddi

180. Which one of the following is a true statement about the lower esophageal sphincter?

(A) It is a true anatomic sphincter
(B) Its resting tension is decreased in achalasia
(C) Its resting tension is increased during pregnancy
(D) It does not respond to sympathetic stimulation
(E) It relaxes during swallowing

181. In contrast to secondary esophageal peristalsis, primary esophageal peristalsis is characterized by which of the following statements?

(A) It does not involve relaxation of the lower esophageal sphincter
(B) It involves contraction of esophageal smooth muscle
(C) It is not influenced by the intrinsic nervous system
(D) It has an oropharyngeal phase
(E) None of the above

182. Absorption of fat-soluble vitamins requires

(A) intrinsic factor
(B) chymotrypsin
(C) pancreatic lipase
(D) pancreatic amylase
(E) none of the above

DIRECTIONS: Each numbered question or incomplete statement below is NEGATIVELY phrased. Select the **one best** lettered response.

183. All the following are correct statements about pancreatic exocrine secretion EXCEPT

(A) bicarbonate-rich fluid is secreted by ductal epithelial cells in response to secretin
(B) secretion of enzymes by acinar cells occurs in response to cholecystokinin
(C) vagotomy augments secretion of enzymes after a meal
(D) secretin and cholecystokinin both act via formation of cyclic nucleotide second messengers
(E) gastrin stimulates both enzyme and bicarbonate secretion

184. All the following are correct statements about salivary secretion EXCEPT

(A) pH goes from acidic to basic as salivary secretory rate increases
(B) salivary secretion is stimulated by increased serum gastrin levels
(C) salivary secretion is stimulated by both parasympathetic and sympathetic neural input
(D) salivary secretions contain organic substances that are bacteriocidal
(E) the concentration of potassium in salivary secretions is greater than that in plasma

185. All the following statements are correct about cholecystokinin (CCK) EXCEPT

(A) CCK is released by fat in the small intestine
(B) CCK increases pancreatic enzyme secretion
(C) CCK contracts gallbladder smooth muscle
(D) CCK contracts sphincter of Oddi smooth muscle
(E) CCK decreases gastric emptying

186. Which one of the following statements about gastric secretory products is NOT correct?

(A) Pepsin is secreted as an inactive proenzyme known as *pepsinogen*
(B) The parietal cell secretes both HCl and intrinsic factor
(C) Pepsin is inactive at a pH of 3 and below
(D) Ionic composition of gastric juice depends upon the rate of secretion
(E) HCl secretion is decreased by drugs that inhibit H^+,K^+-ATPase activity

187. Which one of the following statements about the gastric mucosal barrier is NOT correct?

(A) It limits backflow of H^+ into the gastric mucosal and submucosal areas
(B) It is disrupted by alcohol
(C) It is disrupted by bile salts
(D) It is disrupted by chronic ingestion of aspirin
(E) It is disrupted by vagotomy

188. All the following statements about bile acids are correct EXCEPT

(A) bile acids are secreted as conjugated bile salts by the liver
(B) bile acids are dehydroxylated by intestinal bacteria
(C) bile acids are absorbed in the intestine and return to the liver via the portal vein
(D) bile acids facilitate absorption of fat by emulsifying glycerides
(E) sulfation of bile acids promotes their uptake in the intestine

189. The presence of chyme within the small intestine will lead to all the following EXCEPT

(A) a decrease in the rate of gastric emptying
(B) an increase in the secretion of gastric acid
(C) an increase in intestinal segmentation
(D) contraction of the gallbladder
(E) pancreatic secretion of bicarbonate

190. Bile salts promote absorption of lipids as a result of their ability to do all the following EXCEPT

(A) form micelles, or water-soluble complexes
(B) reduce surface tension of fat particles
(C) increase transit time of lipids in the gut
(D) emulsify fat
(E) stimulate reesterification in the mucosal cells

191. Insulin produces all the following effects EXCEPT

(A) increased utilization of glucose
(B) increased lipolysis
(C) decreased proteolysis
(D) decreased gluconeogenesis
(E) decreased ketogenesis

192. Absorption of fat involves all the following processes EXCEPT

(A) acylation of glycerol-3-phosphate
(B) acylation of mono- and diglycerides
(C) thioesterification of fatty acids
(D) hydrolysis of luminal fat by pancreatic lipase
(E) acidification of luminal contents prior to emulsification

193. The pancreas has both an endocrine and an exocrine function. The nonhormonal substances released by the pancreas serve all the following functions EXCEPT

(A) neutralizing the acid that enters the duodenum
(B) breaking down carbohydrate bonds
(C) breaking down lipids
(D) breaking down proteins
(E) increasing trypsin activity

194. All the following statements concerning normal human pancreatic juice are true EXCEPT

(A) its pH is approximately 8.0
(B) it has a high bicarbonate content
(C) over 1000 mL are secreted per day
(D) it contains cholesterol esterase
(E) its secretion is primarily under neural control

195. Excess fluid loss in the stool (diarrhea) can develop as a consequence of all the following EXCEPT

(A) a decrease in neutral NaCl absorption
(B) bile salts in the colon
(C) fatty acids in the colon
(D) an accumulation of nonabsorbable sugars in the small intestine
(E) a decrease in colonic motility

196. Gastric acid secretion is stimulated by the presence of all the following EXCEPT

(A) acetylcholine
(B) caffeine
(C) gastrin
(D) histamine
(E) norepinephrine

197. The intestinal brush border promotes digestion by all the following EXCEPT

(A) acting as a protective barrier for intestinal epithelium
(B) facilitating movement of intestinal contents
(C) increasing the surface area of the intestinal mucosa
(D) supplying digestive enzymes
(E) supplying specialized transport systems

198. All the following statements about migrating motor complexes (MMCs) in humans are correct EXCEPT

(A) they are correlated with increases in plasma motilin
(B) they are periods of intense contractile activity
(C) they occur only during the interdigestive period
(D) they occur exclusively in the small intestine
(E) they require an intact intrinsic nervous system for coordinated propagation

199. The stimulation of release of pancreatic secretions normally involves all the following EXCEPT

(A) acetylcholine
(B) cholecystokinin
(C) histamine
(D) neural stimulation
(E) secretin

200. In a normal person, all the following circumstances will elicit the enterogastric reflex EXCEPT

(A) increased duodenal pressure
(B) irritation of the small bowel
(C) excessive protein catabolites in the duodenum
(D) acid chyme in the duodenum
(E) pancreatic juice in the duodenum

201. True statements about bile acids include all the following EXCEPT

(A) conjugation of bile acids with glycine or taurine increases the likelihood of formation of micelles
(B) dihydroxy bile acids decrease the absorption of water from the colon
(C) primary bile acids are formed in the liver from cholesterol
(D) secondary bile acids are formed in the small bowel
(E) secretin increases the rate of synthesis of primary bile acids by the liver

202. Intestinal proteolysis is accomplished by all the following EXCEPT

(A) carboxypeptidase
(B) chymotrypsin
(C) elastase
(D) pepsin
(E) trypsin

203. Human bile acids include all the following substances EXCEPT

(A) cholic acid
(B) chenodeoxycholic acid
(C) deoxycholic acid
(D) lithocholic acid
(E) uric acid

Gastrointestinal Physiology

Answers

149. The answer is B. *(Guyton, 8/e, pp 715–716.)* Secretion of gastrin by antral G cells occurs in response to antral distention and certain chemical stimuli, such as amino acids and calcium, but is directly inhibited by the presence of hydrochloric acid in the antrum. This feedback inhibition is important in protecting the gastric mucosa from excessive acid and also in maintaining optimum pH for function of gastric enzymes. Chronic administration of antacid to maintain gastric pH at 7 would abolish this negative feedback control mechanism and thus cause an increase in gastrin secretion.

150. The answer is E. *(Berne, 3/e, pp 640–644. Johnson, pp 470–471.)* In the human, the contractile frequency of the small intestine decreases in an aborad direction. The contractions, which are due to underlying changes in smooth muscle electrical activity called *electrical slow waves*, decrease from approximately 11 per minute in the duodenum to approximately 6 to 7 per minute in the distal ileum. *Segmentation*, the primary motility pattern of the digestive period, is defined as irregular and uncoordinated contraction of the circular muscle layer. This pattern, which develops in response to intestinal wall distention, is determined by activation of preprogrammed neural circuits within the intraluminal myenteric plexus. Elimination of extrinsic input to the bowel wall has little functional effect on bowel motility during the digestive period. Segmentation develops immediately upon the delivery of food into the small intestine and is accompanied by abolishment of the migrating motor complexes characteristic of the interdigestive period.

151. The answer is E. *(Berne, 3/e, pp 633–638.)* The rate of gastric emptying is regulated by stimuli that originate in both the stomach and the proximal small intestine. Distention of the orad stomach elicits an inhibitory vagovagal accommodation reflex that controls intragastric pressure and the emptying of liquids. Distention of the caudad stomach elicits an excitatory vagovagal reflex that results in the trituration of solid food in particles of 1 mm and smaller. Because solids must be liquefied prior to emptying from the stomach, the gastric emptying of liquids begins before the emptying of solids. The actual rate of emptying depends upon neural (enterogastric reflex) and hormonal (enterogastrone) inhibitory feedback from the proximal small bowel. Undigested food residue empties during the interdigestive period in concert with the development of migrating motor complexes.

152. The answer is D. *(Berne, 3/e, pp 707–709.)* Vitamin B_{12} (cobalamin) absorption requires intrinsic factor, a glycoprotein secreted by the parietal cells of the gastric mucosa. The vitamin B_{12}–intrinsic factor complex is emptied from the stomach and propelled along the small intestine to the terminal ileum, where specific transporters located on the enterocyte microvilli bind the vitamin B_{12}–intrinsic factor complex. Binding requires calcium and is optimal at pH 6.6. Absorption is an active transport process.

153. The answer is B. *(Berne, 3/e, pp 664–666. Johnson, pp 458–459, 485–490.)* Gastric acid secretion by the parietal cell occurs in response to excitatory neural (acetylcholine), hormonal (gastrin), and paracrine (histamine) stimuli. Inhibitory feedback regulation of acid output also involves neural (enterogastric reflex), hormonal (enterogastrone), and paracrine (somatostatin) influences. Somatostatis is located in SS cells within the gastric mucosa and is released by hydrogen ions.

154. The answer is D. *(Berne, 3/e, pp 664–669. Johnson, pp 485–492.)* Secretion of hydrochloric acid by the parietal cell occurs in response to neural (vagus nerve), hormonal (gastrin), and paracrine (histamine) stimuli. Acidification of the gastric antrum decreases gastrin release and thereby decreases acid output. Vagotomy and administration of an H_2-receptor antagonist also reduce acid output. Since the amount of acid secretion also depends upon the number of parietal cells present, any disease that results in a decrease in the number of parietal cells (e.g., gastric ulcer disease) will be characterized by a decreased acid output. Conversely, patients with an increased number of parietal cells, as in duodenal ulcer disease, have increased acid secretion.

155. The answer is B. *(Berne, 3/e, pp 615–618, 626.)* Relaxation of gastrointestinal smooth muscle occurs following activation of noradrenergic, noncholinergic (NANC) nerve fibers. Relaxation occurs in response to extrinsic vagal stimulation and stimulation of intrinsic nervous system pathways. Acetylcholine, substance P, and dopamine are excitatory neurotransmitters. Somatostatin is a paracrine secretory product with multiple effects on gastrointestinal function.

156. The answer is C. *(Berne, 3/e, pp 664–668.)* Stimulation of the parietal cell occurs in response to excitatory neural (vagus nerve, acetylcholine), hormonal (gastrin, entero-oxyntin), and paracrine (histamine) influences. Somatostatin is a paracrine secretory product involved in the inhibitory feedback regulation of gastric acid secretion.

157. The answer is A. *(Berne, 3/e, pp 686, 703.)* Diarrhea is defined as the excretion of 200 g or more of water in the stools of an adult during a 24-h period. Cholera, the most severe form of diarrheal disease, produces its effect by increasing salt and water secretion by intestinal crypt cells and by inhibiting salt and water absorption by the villous tip cells of the ileum. Although Na is absorbed from the small intestine by several mechanisms, cholera toxin specifically inhibits neutral NaCl absorption.

158. The answer is D. *(Berne, 3/e, pp 697–703.)* The small intestine and colon absorb approximately 9 to 12 L of fluid per 24-h period, most of which comes from gastrointestinal secretions. Most absorption occurs in the jejunum, with the duodenum serving primarily as the site of osmotic equilibration of chyme. Water absorption is passive and occurs as the direct result of active Na absorption. In contrast to the small intestine, the colon has a limited capacity to absorb water (approximately 3 to 6 L per day).

159. The answer is C. *(Berne, 3/e, pp 697–703.)* Excessive loss of fluid from the gastrointestinal tract can lead to dehydration and, depending upon the origin of the fluid loss, electrolyte and acid-base disturbances. Because the pancreas, liver, ileum, and colon secrete bicarbonate as part of their electrolyte solution, excessive loss leads to metabolic acidosis. In addition, the colon secretes potassium and loss of colonic fluid can lead to hypokalemia. Loss of gastric juice results in hypokalemic, metabolic alkalosis.

160. The answer is C. *(West, 12/e, pp 616–620, 628–630, 632–638.)* Vagal innervation of the gastrointestinal tract extends from the esophagus to the level of the transverse colon. Preganglionic fibers from cell bodies in the medulla synapse with ganglion cells located in the enteric nervous system. Distention-induced contraction of gastrointestinal smooth muscle develops as the result of long (vagovagal) and local (enteric nerves) reflexes. The importance of long versus local reflex pathways varies along the gut. Secondary esophageal peristalsis, intestinal segmentation, and migrating motor complexes are unaffected by vagotomy, whereas caudad stomach peristalsis is decreased but not abolished by vagotomy. Orad stomach accommodation depends exclusively upon an intact vagovagal reflex.

161. The answer is B. *(West, 12/e, pp 610, 637–638.)* Motilin is released during the interdigestive period and is believed to be involved in the propagation of the migrating motor complex. All other gastrointestinal hormones are released during the digestive period and coordinate motor and secretory activities.

162.   The answer is A. *(Berne, 3/e, pp 637–638.)* The rate of gastric emptying is influenced by the intragastric volume and by the physical and chemical composition of the chyme in the small intestine. The initial rate of emptying varies directly with the volume of the meal ingested. Increasing the volume, fat content, acidity, or osmolarity of the lumen of the small intestine elicits inhibitory neural (enterogastric reflex) and hormonal (enterogastrone) feedback mechanisms.

163.   The answer is B. *(Berne, 3/e, pp 666–668.)* Secretion of acid occurs because of the complex interaction of neural, hormonal, and paracrine stimuli. The predominant excitatory neural input occurs via the vagus nerve. When vagal input is removed, secretion of acid is decreased. Because the cephalic phase of secretion of acid is mediated exclusively by the vagus nerve, it will be the most affected by vagotomy. Secretion of acid will continue during the other phases (although it will be reduced) because of the other pathways for stimulation.

164.   The answer is A. *(Berne, 3/e, pp 633–634. Johnson, pp 467–468.)* Increases in intragastric volume normally are not associated with large increases in intragastric pressure because of distention-mediated activation of a vagovagal inhibitory reflex, the accommodation reflex. The reflex is a property of the proximal stomach only and counterbalances the stretch-induced myogenic contraction of the gastric smooth muscle. *Peristalsis, trituration* (grinding), and *retropulsion* (mixing) are terms referring to the contractile activity and functions of the distal stomach. Segmentation is the primary contractile pattern of the small intestine during the digestive period.

165.   The answer is A. *(Guyton, 8/e, p 718.)* Liberation of the enzyme enteropeptidase (enterokinase) from the duodenal mucosal cells causes the inactive trypsinogen to be converted to the active form, trypsin. Enteropeptidase contains 41 percent polysaccharide. It is this high level of polysaccharide that is responsible for the fact that enteropeptidase itself is not digested. Trypsin is responsible for the conversion of chymotrypsinogens and other proenzymes into their active forms.

166.   The answer is D. *(Berne, 3/e, pp 697–701.)* Absorption of sodium is the primary absorptive event in the small intestine. Absorption of Na^+ is necessary for absorption of water and other electrolytes. Although multiple pathways exist for the absorption of Na^+, neutral absorption is the major mechanism. Neutral absorption may occur in two ways: Na^+ cotransported with Cl^- or in exchange for H^+ ions.

167. The answer is A. *(Berne, 3/e, pp 660–662. Ganong, 16/e, pp 447–449.)* Secretion of acid by gastric parietal (oxyntic) cells involves stimulation of adenyl cyclase and cyclic AMP–mediated stimulation of the active transport of chloride and potassium-hydrogen ion exchange. Neither gastrin nor vagal stimulation activates adenyl cyclase directly; both depend on concomitant release of histamine and histamine-induced activation of adenyl cyclase. Blockade of histamine H_2 receptors by drugs such as cimetidine thus inhibits both gastrin-induced and vagally mediated secretion of acid.

168. The answer is B. *(Guyton, 8/e, p 722.)* Although several intestinal hormones, including gastrin, cause contraction of the gallbladder, the principal mechanism involved is stimulation by the hormone cholecystokinin (CCK). CCK is elaborated in the duodenum in response to food. It supplements the action of secretin to produce alkaline pancreatic juice and retards gastric emptying. CCK is also thought to be associated with secretin in promoting contraction of the pyloric sphincter.

169. The answer is E. *(Guyton, 8/e, pp 705–707.)* Mass movements (strong peristalsis) in the colon occur about two to three times per day. They are initiated and continued by Auerbach's plexus and are independent of any extrinsic forces or innervation. At least three mass movements are usually required for the colonic contents to reach the rectum. Meissner's plexus is submucosal and has a principally sensory function.

170. The answer is D. *(Berne, 3/e, pp 710–713.)* Triglycerides are hydrolyzed to monoglycerides and taken into mucosal cells. If the fatty acids are short chains (less than 10 to 12 carbon atoms), they are extruded in the form of free fatty acids into the portal blood. If the fatty acids are long chains, they are extruded in the form of chylomicrons into the lymphatic system. Chylomicrons represent triglycerides and esters of cholesterol that have been invested in the intestinal mucosa with a coating of phospholipid, protein, and cholesterol.

171. The answer is B. *(West, 12/e, pp 682–684.)* Unconjugated bilirubin, which is a breakdown product of the heme ring of hemoglobin, is taken up from plasma by the liver, conjugated with glucuronic acid, and released via the bile duct into the gastrointestinal tract. Under normal conditions, some conjugated bilirubin is reabsorbed by the intestine. The kidney clears only conjugated bilirubin. Thus, acute obstruction of the bile duct does not affect the rate of hepatic conjugation of bilirubin but does result in a "backup" of conjugated bilirubin in plasma and in its eventual clearance by the kidney.

172. The answer is C. *(Guyton, 8/e, pp 735, 742.)* The digestive tract normally contains about 150 to 200 mL of gas, most of which is in the colon, with approximately 50 mL in the stomach. Most of the gas in the stomach is derived from air swallowed during eating or in periods of anxiety. Gas is produced in the small intestine by interaction of gastric acid and bicarbonate in the intestinal and pancreatic secretions but does not accumulate because it is either reabsorbed or quickly passed into the colon. Gas within the colon is derived primarily from fermentation of undigested material by intestinal bacteria to produce CO_2, H_2, and methane. The amount of gas varies markedly from one person to another and is influenced by diet; e.g., ingestion of large amounts of beans, which contain undigestible carbohydrates in their hulls, will increase gas formation by intestinal bacteria. Diffusion of gas from the blood to the intestinal lumen is responsible for the N_2 present in intestinal gas and is influenced by the atmospheric pressure.

173. The answer is D. *(Berne, 3/e, pp 633–634, 658–659, 667.)* The distal stomach, which includes the antrum and the pyloric sphincter, is involved in the regulation of the gastric emptying of solids and in the regulation of secretion of acid. Antral peristaltic contractions are necessary for the adequate trituration of solids. The pyloric sphincter serves to limit the flow of solids out of the stomach until the particles are of a small enough size to be suspended in the liquid component of the meal. Removal of the antrum and the sphincter will increase the rate of gastric emptying because the resistance to flow of large particles will be removed. Secretion of acid will be decreased because of the loss of gastrin, which is normally secreted by the G cells of the antrum. Gastric compliance is a property of the proximal stomach.

174. The answer is B. *(Berne, 3/e, pp 678–679, 684, 705–706, 711–714.)* The terminal ileum contains specialized cells responsible for the absorption of primary and secondary bile salts by active transport. Bile salts are necessary for adequate digestion and absorption of fat. In the absence of the terminal ileum there will be an increase in the amounts of bile acids and fatty acids delivered to the colon. Fats and bile salts in the colon increase the water content of the feces by promoting the influx (secretion) of water into the lumen of the colon. Amino acids are absorbed in the jejunum. Iron is primarily absorbed in the duodenum.

175. The answer is E. *(West, 12/e, pp 704–705.)* Several vitamins—including vitamin K, several of the B complex, and folic acid—can be synthesized by intestinal bacteria. However, in humans, only folic acid so synthesized is absorbed by the host. Dietary intake of the other vitamins is necessary.

176. The answer is D. *(Johnson, pp 519–521.)* The parietal cells of the gastric mucosa secrete acid in response to gastrin, acetylcholine, and histamine stimulation. Two different types of histamine receptors, H_1 and H_2, have been identified in the body. Gastric acid secretion is mediated by H_2 receptors, which are selectively inhibited by cimetidine, whereas antihistamines that are used clinically to treat the nasal and sinus congestion in allergic reactions act at H_1 receptors. Acid secretion is a process that requires energy for the active transport of H^+ and Cl^- and utilizes CO_2. The following net reaction illustrates the process, but does not describe the actual sequence of chemical reactions:

$$CO_2 + H_2O + NaCl \rightarrow HCl + NaHCO_3$$

Chief cells contain zymogen granules and secrete pepsinogens.

177. The answer is A. *(Berne, 3/e, pp 697–701.)* The major route of absorption of sodium in the colon is electrogenic transport. Because of the "tight" nature of the tight junctions that connect cells in the colon, a relatively large potential difference exists between the mucosal (negative) and serosal (positive) surfaces of the absorptive cells. This electrical difference favors the net secretion of K^+ into the lumen. The amounts of absorption of Na^+ and secretion of K^+ can be affected by changes in levels of aldosterone. Secretion of HCO_3^- occurs in exchange for absorption of Cl^-. No counterbalancing cation exchange pumps are present in the colon. Bile acids in the colon would hold water in the colon.

178. The answer is D. *(Johnson, pp 503–505.)* Contraction of the gallbladder and relaxation of the sphincter of Oddi at the junction of the common bile duct and duodenum are necessary for delivery of bile into the duodenum. These muscular actions are under both hormonal and neural control. Cholecystokinin is a peptide secreted by the duodenal mucosa in response to entry of food, especially fatty acids and amino acids. The hormone acts to promote gallbladder contraction and probably to relax the sphincter of Oddi; it also elicits secretion of enzyme-rich pancreatic juice. Vagal stimulation, which is cholinergically mediated and blocked by atropine, also promotes gallbladder contraction.

179. The answer is C. *(Berne, 3/e, pp 455–457.)* Acidification of the small intestine causes release of the hormone secretin. Secretin is the primary stimulus for pancreatic secretion of water and bicarbonate. In addition secretin may serve as an enterogastrone, i.e., a hormone involved in the inhibitory feedback regulation of gastric function. Cholecystokinin (CCK) is the hormone responsible for contraction of the gallbladder and relaxation of the sphincter of Oddi.

180. The answer is E. *(Ganong, 16/e, pp 445–446.)* There is no discrete muscular band at the gastroesophageal junction that forms an anatomic lower esophageal sphincter (LES). Intraluminal pressure measurements have demonstrated a segment 4 to 6 cm in length beginning about 2 cm above the diaphragm in which intraluminal pressure is increased by an increase in muscle tone so that this segment functions as a physiologic sphincter. Tonic activity of this sphincter between meals prevents reflux of acidic gastric contents into the esophagus, whose squamous mucosa lacks a protective mucous coating. During swallowing, this segment relaxes to permit passage of the swallowed material into the stomach. The esophagus is innervated by both sympathetic and parasympathetic divisions of the autonomic system. In achalasia, the tension in the lower esophageal sphincter is increased by pathologic changes in the vagal fibers, so that food accumulates in the esophagus, which becomes markedly dilated. During pregnancy, the resting tension in the lower esophageal sphincter is decreased. This is a contributing factor in the increase in acid reflux during pregnancy.

181. The answer is D. *(Berne, 3/e, pp 627–633.)* The term *primary esophageal peristalsis* denotes that swallowing has been elicited as a consequence of activation of the "swallowing centers" in the medulla. The event involves not only esophageal peristalsis and relaxation of the lower esophageal sphincter (LES), but also the transit of food through the pharyngeal region. It is initiated via the vagus nerve. Secondary esophageal peristalsis is a localized esophageal response to irritation or distention that results in a peristaltic contraction and relaxation of the LES. Both primary and secondary esophageal peristalsis involve the intrinsic nervous system.

182. The answer is C. *(Berne, 3/e, pp 709–715.)* Absorption of the fat-soluble vitamins (A, D, E, and K) is diminished if there is a lack of bile or pancreatic lipase. Lipase is required to produce monoglycerides that, in combination with bile salts, make it possible to bring the fat-soluble vitamins close to the mucosal cell surface for absorption. With the exception of vitamin B_{12}, which is absorbed bound to intrinsic factor in the ileum, vitamins are absorbed chiefly in the upper small intestine.

183. The answer is C. *(Guyton, 8/e, pp 718–720.)* Cholecystokinin released in response to the presence of amino acids and peptides in the duodenum is the major stimulant of enzyme secretion by pancreatic acinar cells and also weakly stimulates secretion of bicarbonate-rich fluid by ductal epithelial cells. Parasympathetic stimulation via the vagus is also a major stimulant of enzyme secretion. Thus, vagotomy drastically reduces enzyme secretion after a meal. The major stimulant for bicarbonate secretion is secretin, which is released from the duodenum in response to acidification of the luminal contents. Both cholecystokinin and secretin act by stimulating the formation of cyclic nucleotide second messengers—cyclic AMP in the case of secretin and cyclic GMP in the case of cholecystokinin. Gastrin can mimic the effects of cholecystokinin because both have the same C terminal amino acid sequence.

184. The answer is B. *(Ganong, 16/e, pp 444–445. Johnson, pp 477–481.)* Bicarbonate is present in saliva; its concentration increases with increased salivary flow, thereby producing an increasingly alkaline fluid. The control of salivary secretion is exclusively neural and involves both parasympathetic cholinergic nerves and sympathetic adrenergic nerves. Stimulation of salivary secretion produces a fluid high in potassium and containing lysozymes capable of destroying certain bacteria, including *Staphylococcus, Proteus*, and *Streptococcus*.

185. The answer is D. *(Berne, 3/e, pp 638, 679–685. Johnson, pp 455–457.)* Cholecystokinin (CCK) is the principal hormone responsible for gallbladder emptying and pancreatic enzyme secretion. Gallbladder emptying occurs as a result of contraction of gallbladder smooth muscle and relaxation of the sphincter of Oddi. Released in response to the delivery of fat into the proximal small bowel, CCK also contributes to the inhibitory feedback regulation of gastric emptying.

186. The answer is C. *(Berne, 3/e, pp 658–663.)* Gastric juice is a collection of organic and inorganic products, the exact composition of which depends upon the secretory rate. Parietal cells secrete both HCl and intrinsic factor. HCl secretion is an active transport process mediated via an H^+,K^+-ATPase enzyme. The proteolytic enzyme pepsin is secreted as the proenzyme pepsinogen by the gastric chief cells. Conversion of pepsinogen to pepsin occurs at pHs of 5.5 and lower.

187. The answer is E. *(Berne, 3/e, pp 663–664.)* The gastric mucosal barrier refers to the ability of the mucosal lining of the stomach to resist the corrosive effects of HCl. Backflow of hydrogen ions into the submucosa is limited by the secretion of bicarbonate and mucus, by the characteristics of mucosal blood flow, and by the integrity of the mucosal surface of the cells facing the lumen of the stomach. The local production of prostaglandins is believed to promote the integrity of the barrier.

Disruption of the mucosal barrier can be caused by exposure of the gastric mucosa to factors that physically disrupt the barrier (e.g., alcohol, bile salts) or that decrease local prostaglandin production (aspirin). The vagus nerve has no effect on the integrity of the mucosal barrier.

188.   The answer is E. *(Guyton, 8/e, pp 720–723.)* Primary bile acids are synthesized from cholesterol in the liver by the addition of hydroxyl and carboxyl groups and are secreted as amide conjugates with either taurine or glycine. Dehydroxylation of these compounds by intestinal bacteria forms secondary bile acids. Both primary and secondary bile acids are reabsorbed primarily by active transport in the ileum and return to the liver via the portal vein, where they are reutilized and secreted in the bile. Because they possess both hydrophobic and hydrophilic properties, bile acids and their salts accumulate at lipid-water interfaces and thus emulsify dietary fat and promote its hydrolysis. Sulfation of bile acids occurs in the liver. Since sulfated bile acids are not reabsorbed in the ileum, this process is a major route for excretion of these compounds in the feces.

189.   The answer is B. *(Berne, 3/e, pp 637–638, 667–668, 673–676, 683–684.)* Food in the small intestine elicits a number of neurally and hormonally mediated reflexes that govern the activity of the GI tract. Cholecystokinin (CCK) and secretin act to stimulate secretion of pancreatic enzymes and HCO_3^-, while at the same time they play a role in the inhibitory feedback regulation of gastric emptying and secretion of acid. The distention caused by the presence of food activates a complex series of reflexes mediated by the intrinsic nervous system; these reflexes increase the segmental contractile pattern of the bowel.

190.   The answer is C. *(Berne, 3/e, pp 678–680, 710–713. Ganong, 16/e, pp 455–456.)* Bile salts combine with lipids to form micelles. Micelles are water-soluble complexes that are more easily absorbed than uncombined lipids, which are hydrophobic. Prior to micelle formation, bile salts exercise an emulsifying action on fat particles that involves a reduction in surface tension of such particles. Emulsification of fat particles, in which fatty acids and glycerides also participate, facilitates digestion and absorption. Reesterification of fatty acids in the mucosal cells — another prerequisite for absorption — also is stimulated by bile salts.

191.   The answer is B. *(Berne, 3/e, pp 305–312.)* The main function of insulin is to stimulate anabolic reactions involving carbohydrates, fats, proteins, and nucleic acids. Therefore, insulin increases the utilization of glucose while stimulating lipogenesis and proteogenesis. By promoting utilization of glucose in cells, insulin diminishes the need for gluconeogenesis and ketogenesis.

192. The answer is E. *(Berne, 3/e, pp 710–713.)* Absorption of fat occurs primarily in the duodenum and proximal jejunum and initially involves the formation of micelles by bile salts and phospholipids, fatty acids, and glycerides in order to solubilize the water-insoluble fat. Micelle formation is enhanced by the alkalinization of luminal contents by pancreatic and biliary secretions, a process that favors dissociation of fatty acids and improves their water solubility and interactions with other micellar components. Pancreatic lipase acts on micelles, releasing fatty acids and 2-monoglycerides that are taken up into mucosal cells. Fatty acids are then activated to acyl CoA thioesters and incorporated into phospholipids and triglycerides. They are released into the lymph as chylomicrons.

193. The answer is E. *(Guyton, 8/e, pp 718–719.)* The pancreas releases several enzymes that aid in the digestion of fat, protein, and carbohydrate and that demonstrate optimal activity above pH 7.0. Pancreatic secretions are rich in HCO_3^- and thus neutralize acid entering the duodenum. Trypsin is a proteolytic enzyme that is released in the intestinal lumen from its inactive precursor, trypsinogen, which is formed in the pancreas. Activation of trypsin within the pancreas is prevented by the pancreatic secretion of a trypsin inhibitor, which, by blocking the activation of trypsin, prevents autodigestion.

194. The answer is E. *(Ganong, 16/e, pp 452–453. Guyton, 8/e, pp 718–719.)* Pancreatic juice is rich in bicarbonate and, having a pH of about 8.0, neutralizes gastric acid entering the duodenum. It is secreted at the rate of 1 to 2 L per day and contains several proteolytic enzymes of digestion, such as trypsin and elastase, as well as enzymes of fat and carbohydrate digestion. Pancreatic exocrine secretion is controlled primarily by the hormones secretin and cholecystokinin, which are secreted by cells in the small intestinal mucosa.

195. The answer is E. *(Berne, 3/e, pp 697–301.)* Fluid balance in the small intestine and the colon is the summation of factors that favor absorption and those that favor secretion. For example, bile salts and fatty acids in the colon decrease absorption of water while at the same time they increase the flow of water into the lumen. The net result is excess fluid loss. Similarly, a decrease in the amount of water absorbed as a result of a decrease in neutral NaCl absorption in the small intestine or as the result of the increased presence of osmotic particles (nonabsorbable) in the small intestine may lead to diarrhea if the increased volume presented to the colon exceeds the maximal daily absorptive capacity of the colon (5 L per day).

196. The answer is E. *(Ganong, 16/e, pp 447–451.)* Gastric acid secretion is regulated by both neural and local stimuli. The cephalic phase, which occurs in response to smell or sight of food, is mediated by cholinergic fibers of the vagus nerve that act either directly on parietal cells or stimulate gastrin release from G cells in the gastric mucosa. Gastrin is the major hormonal promoter of gastric acid secretion and is released in response to the presence of protein in the gastric lumen and in response to the hormone bombesin and to cholinergic or beta-adrenergic stimulation. (Norepinephrine is primarily alpha-adrenergic.) Histamine is a potent stimulus for secretion of acid that is produced locally in the stomach. Some effects of stimuli other than those of histamine appear to be mediated in part by histamine since they are partially blocked by cimetidine, a selective histamine H_2-receptor antagonist that has, to a large extent, replaced surgery in the management of peptic ulcer disease. Caffeine and alcohol stimulate acid secretion by direct action on the mucosa.

197. The answer is B. *(Johnson, pp 507–510.)* The brush border on the luminal surface of the small intestine is formed by (1) microvilli on the surface of each epithelial cell and (2) an amorphous layer rich in neutral and amino sugars known as the glycocalyx, which forms a protective barrier. Within the brush border are numerous enzymes for hydrolysis of disaccharides, peptides, and nucleic acids, as well as specialized transport systems. The primary function of the brush border is to enhance absorption by increasing the surface area for transport. It has no role in movement of intestinal contents.

198. The answer is D. *(Berne, 3/e, pp 642–644.)* Migrating motor complexes (MMCs) are periods of intense electrical and contractile activity that occur at intervals in the interdigestive period. In humans, MMCs occur every 75 to 90 min and appear to involve both a neural input via the intrinsic nervous system and a hormonal input (motilin). The plasma level of motilin rises in concert with the generation of the MMC. Although they were originally described as occurring only in the small intestine, it is now well known that MMCs are present in the stomach and perhaps in the esophagus.

199. The answer is C. *(Berne, 3/e, pp 668–675.)* Pancreatic secretion is under both neural and hormonal control. Neural control is by way of the vagus nerve and involves acetylcholine-mediated increases in enzymatic secretion. Hormonal stimulation of the pancreas is due to secretin, which increases output of water and bicarbonate, and cholecystokinin, which increases enzymatic output. Histamine plays a role in the regulation of secretion of gastric acid.

200. The answer is E. *(Guyton, 8/e, pp 702–703.)* The enterogastric reflex inhibits the activity of the pyloric pump and slows gastric emptying. It is mediated primarily by afferent fibers of the vagus nerve that transmit impulses to nuclei in the brainstem. Some direct transmission of impulses via the myenteric plexus also occurs. The reflex is elicited by irritation of the small bowel, increased duodenal pressure, excessive protein catabolites in the duodenum, or the presence of acid chyme in that part of the small intestine (pancreatic juice is alkaline). It acts to slow gastric emptying, thus permitting sufficient time for digestion and absorption of duodenal contents.

201. The answer is E. *(Berne, 3/e, pp 679–683.)* The conversion of cholesterol to primary bile acids takes place in the liver. Secondary bile acids are formed in the small intestine as a consequence of bacterial alteration of the primary bile acids. In order for both the primary and the secondary bile acids to be effective in promoting the digestion and absorption of fats, it is necessary that they form aggregates called *micelles.* Conjugation of the bile salts with glycine or taurine greatly enhances the probability of formation of micelles. Secretin is responsible for stimulation of the bile acid–independent fraction of bile. The presence of any osmotically active particles in the colon holds water in the stool and decreases water absorption.

202. The answer is D. *(Johnson, pp 508, 512–513.)* Protein digestion begins with the action of pepsins in the stomach. Because pepsins require a pH of 1.6 to 3.2, they are rendered inactive when they reach the more alkaline environment of the duodenum. Trypsin, chymotrypsin, elastase, and carboxypeptidase all are proteolytic enzymes that are active in the intestine.

203. The answer is E. *(Berne, 3/e, pp 678–681.)* Cholic, chenodeoxycholic, deoxycholic, and lithocholic acids all have been isolated from human bile. The sodium and potassium salts of these acids (bile salts) are important in emulsification and the formation of micelles for fat absorption. They also activate intestinal lipases and stimulate glycerol synthesis and reesterification of fatty acids.

Respiratory Physiology

DIRECTIONS: Each question below contains five suggested responses. Select the **one best** response to each question.

204. The basic respiratory rhythm is generated by the

(A) apneustic center
(B) nucleus parabrachialis
(C) dorsal medulla
(D) pneumotaxic center
(E) cerebrum

205. At the end of a quiet inspiration, intraalveolar pressure is normally

(A) -40 cmH$_2$0
(B) -4 cmH$_2$0
(C) 0 cm H$_2$0
(D) $+4$ cmH$_2$0
(E) $+40$ cmH$_2$0

Questions 206–208

The diagram below represents a spirometry tracing illustrating the changes in lung volume that occurred when a subject inhaled maximally and then rapidly exhaled as much gas as possible.

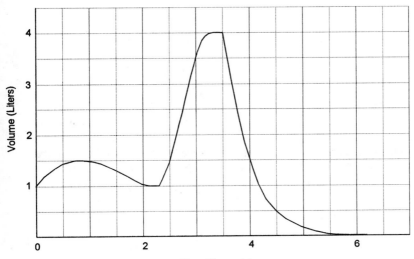

206. If the patient's total lung capacity is 6 L, what is the functional residual capacity?

(A) 1 L
(B) 2 L
(C) 3 L
(D) 4 L
(E) 5 L

207. What is the FEV$_1$?

(A) 1.5 L
(B) 2.5 L
(C) 3.5 L
(D) 4.5 L
(E) 5.5 L

208. What is the inspiratory capacity?

(A) 1.0 L
(B) 1.5 L
(C) 2.0 L
(D) 2.5 L
(E) 3.0 L

209. A man ascends to an altitude at which the atmospheric pressure is 400 mmHg. If he reduces his PA$_{CO_2}$ to 30 mmHg by hyperventilating, his PA$_{O_2}$ will be closest to

(A) 95 mmHg
(B) 75 mmHg
(C) 55 mmHg
(D) 45 mmHg
(E) 35 mmHg

210. After performing a forced vital capacity test, a woman begins to breathe into a 12 L spirometer containing 10% helium. After several minutes, the helium concentration in the spirometer falls to 8.5%. If her vital capacity is 5 L, what is her total lung capacity?

(A) 3 L
(B) 5 L
(C) 7 L
(D) 9 L
(E) 11 L

211. Which of the following lung volumes will change by the greatest amount when a normal person moves from a standing to a supine position?

(A) Functional residual capacity
(B) Residual volume
(C) Total lung capacity
(D) Vital capacity
(E) Tidal volume

Questions 212–213

212. A woman has a respiratory rate of 18, a tidal volume of 350 mL, and a dead space of 100 mL. What is her alveolar ventilation?

(A) 4.0 L
(B) 4.5 L
(C) 5.0 L
(D) 5.5 L
(E) 6.0 L

213. This woman has a normal PA_{CO_2}. If she increases her tidal volume by 75 mL, her PA_{CO_2} will become approximately

(A) 15 mmHg
(B) 20 mmHg
(C) 25 mmHg
(D) 30 mmHg
(E) 35 mmHg

Questions 214–215

The diagram below illustrates the intrapleural pressure generated by a patient who exhales forcefully after a maximal inhalation.

214. If the intrapleural pressure at the end of inspiration is 10 cmH$_2$O and the intrapleural pressure during expiration is 30 cmH$_2$O, the equal pressure point will be closest to point

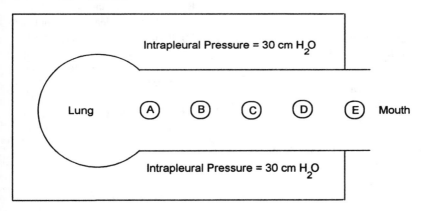

(A) A
(B) B
(C) C
(D) D
(E) E

215. The equal pressure point would be most likely to move closer to the mouth with an increase in

(A) airway resistance
(B) lung compliance
(C) lung volume
(D) expiratory effort
(E) airway smooth muscle tone

216. Which one of the following would increase in obstructive but not in restrictive lung disease?

(A) Vital capacity
(B) Maximum breathing capacity
(C) FEV_1
(D) Functional residual capacity
(E) Breathing frequency

217. During the early stages of an asthmatic attack,

(A) arterial carbon dioxide tension decreases
(B) the equal pressure point moves toward the mouth
(C) lung compliance increases
(D) tidal volume decreases
(E) arterial oxygen tension increases

218. Which one of the following will decrease in a person with ventilation-perfusion $(\dot{V}/\dot{Q})$ abnormalities?

(A) Anion gap
(B) Arterial pH
(C) Arterial carbon dioxide tension
(D) Alveolar-arterial (A-a) gradient for oxygen
(E) Alveolar ventilation

219. Which one of the following is higher at the apex of the lung than at the base when a person is standing?

(A) $\dot{V}/\dot{Q}$ ratio
(B) Blood flow
(C) Ventilation
(D) Pa_{CO_2}
(E) Lung compliance

220. Providing oxygen to a patient with chronic obstructive pulmonary disease (COPD) may cause a decrease in ventilation. Which one of the following statements best explains this observation?

(A) Mucous secretion increases
(B) Airway resistance increases
(C) Physiologic dead space increases
(D) Peripheral chemoreceptor activity decreases
(E) Diffusing capacity for oxygen decreases

221. Very small particles are removed from the respiratory system by

(A) bulk flow
(B) diffusion
(C) expectoration
(D) phagocytosis
(E) ciliary transport

222. Low arterial oxygen tension and content is most likely to be observed during

(A) hyperventilation
(B) fever
(C) anemia
(D) carbon monoxide poisoning
(E) respiratory acidosis

223. The bulk of CO_2 is transported in arterial blood as

(A) dissolved CO_2
(B) carbonic acid
(C) carbaminohemoglobin
(D) bicarbonate
(E) carboxyhemoglobin

224. In the diagram of a human airway below, gas exchange occurs in

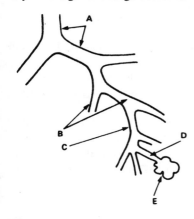

(A) E
(B) E and D
(C) D, C, and B
(D) E, D, C, and B
(E) E, D, C, B, and A

225. The partial pressure of oxygen in dry air (21% O_2) inhaled by divers at a depth of 100 feet below sea level (4 atmospheres) is approximately

(A) 160 mmHg
(B) 320 mmHg
(C) 640 mmHg
(D) 1280 mmHg
(E) none of the above

226. A patient is on a ventilator adjusted for a tidal volume of 1 L at a frequency of 10/min. If the patient's anatomic dead space is 200 mL and the machine's dead space 50 mL, the alveolar ventilation is

(A) 10 L/min
(B) 8.5 L/min
(C) 7.5 L/min
(D) 5 L/min
(E) not determinable from the information given

227. Two healthy women with identical tidal volumes and respiratory rates are subjected to spirometry and blood gas measurements. Subject A doubles her tidal volume and decreases her respiratory rate to one-half of baseline. Subject B decreases her tidal volume to one-half of baseline and doubles her respiratory rate. Which of the following statements about the resulting alveolar ventilation in the two women is true?

(A) Alveolar ventilation is unchanged in both subjects
(B) Alveolar ventilation increases in both subjects
(C) Alveolar ventilation decreases in both subjects
(D) Alveolar ventilation increases in subject A and decreases in subject B
(E) Alveolar ventilation decreases in subject A and increases in subject B

228. The concentration of CO_2 is lowest in

(A) the anatomic dead space at end inspiration
(B) the anatomic dead space at end expiration
(C) the alveoli at end inspiration
(D) the alveoli at end expiration
(E) the blood in the pulmonary veins

229. Peripheral and central chemoreceptors may both contribute to the increased ventilation that occurs as a result of

(A) a decrease in arterial oxygen content
(B) a decrease in arterial blood pressure
(C) an increase in arterial carbon dioxide tension
(D) a decrease in arterial oxygen tension
(E) an increase in arterial pH

230. Complete transection of the brainstem above the pons would

(A) result in cessation of all breathing movements
(B) prevent any voluntary holding of breath
(C) prevent the central chemoreceptors from exerting any control over ventilation
(D) prevent the peripheral chemoreceptors from exerting any control over ventilation
(E) abolish the Hering-Breuer reflex

Questions 231–232

The diagram below illustrates the change in intrapleural pressure during a single breath.

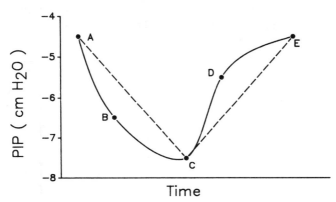

231. At which point on the diagram is inspiratory airflow the greatest?

(A) A
(B) B
(C) C
(D) D
(E) E

232. At which point on the diagram is lung volume the greatest?

(A) A
(B) B
(C) C
(D) D
(E) E

233. The water vapor pressure of alveolar gas at a barometric pressure of 380 mmHg is

(A) 23.5 mmHg
(B) 47.0 mmHg
(C) 76.0 mmHg
(D) 94.0 mmHg
(E) 105.0 mmHg

234. A deficiency of pulmonary surfactant would

(A) decrease surface tension in the alveoli
(B) decrease the change in intrapleural pressure required to achieve a given tidal volume
(C) decrease lung compliance
(D) decrease the work of breathing
(E) increase functional residual capacity (FRC)

Questions 235–236

Measurement of the closing volume is a sensitive test of airway disease. A patient expires to residual volume and then inspires to total lung volume. At the beginning of this inspiration, a small quantity of insoluble inert tracer gas (helium) is injected into the inspired gas. The patient then expires to residual volume and the curve appearing below is produced.

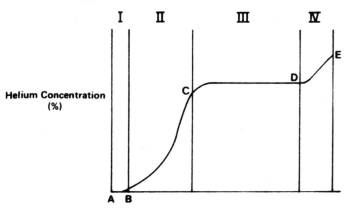

235. Closing volume is measured at point

(A) A
(B) B
(C) C
(D) D
(E) E

236. Closing volume is normally what percentage of vital capacity?

(A) Ten percent in young persons and it increases with age
(B) Ten percent in young persons and it decreases with age
(C) Forty percent in young persons and it increases with age
(D) Forty percent in young persons and it decreases with age
(E) Ninety percent

237. The following data were obtained during a pulmonary function test: fraction of CO_2 in mixed expired gas $(FE_{CO_2}) = 3.0\%$; fraction of CO_2 in alveolar gas $(FA_{CO_2}) = 4.5\%$; tidal volume $(V_T) = 450$ mL (BTPS); and frequency $= 10$ breaths per minute. The volume of the physiologic dead space (V_D) is

(A) 100 mL
(B) 150 mL
(C) 225 mL
(D) 750 mL
(E) 1500 mL

238. A man breathing room air at sea level has an alveolar ventilation of 2 L/min. The blood gases show a Pa_{CO_2} of 48 mmHg and a Pa_{O_2} of 70 mmHg. The alveolar oxygen tension (PA_{O_2}) is

(A) 150 mmHg
(B) 110 mmHg
(C) 100 mmHg
(D) 90 mmHg
(E) 60 mmHg

239. A young skier with normal pulmonary function (minute volume 4L; pulmonary blood flow 5 L/min) who is recovering from a tibial fracture suddenly develops right-sided chest pain and tachypnea. Embolic occlusion of the right pulmonary artery is suspected. The diagnosis would be immediately confirmed by which of the following tracheal gas measurements?

	P_{O_2} (mmHg)	P_{CO_2} (mmHg)
(A)	125	60
(B)	125	20
(C)	100	40
(D)	80	20
(E)	80	60

240. Measurement of the lecithin-sphingomyelin (L-S) ratio in amniotic fluid assesses

(A) the placenta's ability to oxygenate the fetus
(B) fetal adrenal function
(C) fetal kidney development
(D) fetal brain development
(E) fetal lung maturity

241. When the respiratory muscles are relaxed, the lungs are at

(A) residual volume (RV)
(B) expiratory reserve volume (ERV)
(C) functional residual capacity (FRC)
(D) inspiratory reserve volume (IRV)
(E) total lung capacity (TLC)

242. Which one of the following is the most likely cause of a high arterial P_{CO_2}?

(A) Increased metabolic activity
(B) Increased alveolar dead space
(C) Depressed medullary respiratory centers
(D) Alveolar capillary block
(E) Increased alveolar ventilation

243. The resistance of the large- and medium-sized airways as a percentage of the total airway resistance is approximately

(A) 10 percent
(B) 20 percent
(C) 40 percent
(D) 60 percent
(E) 80 percent

244. Pulmonary vascular resistance increases

(A) as the lung volume approaches TLC
(B) as the lung volume approaches FRC
(C) as the cardiac output increases
(D) as pulmonary artery pressure increases
(E) as left atrial pressure increases

245. Which of the following would normally be found to be less in the fetus than in the mother?

(A) Pa_{CO_2}
(B) Pulmonary vascular resistance
(C) Affinity of hemoglobin for oxygen
(D) Pa_{O_2}
(E) Arterial hydrogen ion concentration

246. During a forced expiration, actively contracting muscles include the

(A) sternocleidomastoid
(B) diaphragm
(C) abdominal muscles
(D) external intercostals
(E) scalene

247. During moderate aerobic exercise,

(A) Pa_{O_2} increases
(B) Pa_{CO_2} decreases
(C) arterial pH decreases
(D) alveolar ventilation increases
(E) blood lactate level increases

248. Reduction of functional hemoglobin associated with anemia, methemoglobinemia, or carbon monoxide poisoning does not produce hyperpnea because the

(A) blood flow to the carotid body is decreased
(B) total arterial oxygen content is maintained within the normal range
(C) carotid body chemoreceptors are stimulated
(D) central chemoreceptors are stimulated
(E) P_{O_2} of arterial blood is normal

249. Pulmonary alveoli are kept dry by factors that include the

(A) phagocytic activity of alveolar macrophages
(B) negative interstitial fluid pressure
(C) low vapor pressure of water in inspired air
(D) secretion of surfactant
(E) tight junctions between the alveolar capillary endothelial cells

250. As the P_{CO_2} of the venous blood increases,

(A) the concentration of HCO_3^- decreases
(B) the concentration of H^+ in the red cell decreases
(C) the volume of the red cell increases
(D) the affinity of the hemoglobin for O_2 increases
(E) the amount of chloride in the red cell decreases

251. The percentage of hemoglobin saturated with oxygen will increase if

(A) the arterial P_{CO_2} is increased
(B) the hemoglobin concentration is increased
(C) the temperature is increased
(D) the arterial P_{O_2} is increased
(E) the arterial pH is decreased

252. Which of the following will return toward normal during acclimatization to high altitude?

(A) Arterial hydrogen ion concentration
(B) Arterial carbon dioxide tension
(C) Arterial bicarbonate ion concentration
(D) Arterial hemoglobin concentration
(E) Alveolar ventilation

253. Pulmonary compliance is characterized by which of the following statements?

(A) It decreases with advancing age
(B) It is inversely related to the elastic recoil properties of the lung
(C) It increases in patients with pulmonary edema
(D) It is equivalent to $\Delta P/\Delta V$
(E) It increases when there is a deficiency of surfactant

254. The activity of the central chemoreceptors is stimulated by

(A) an increase in the P_{CO_2} of blood flowing through the brain
(B) a decrease in the P_{O_2} of blood flowing through the brain
(C) a decrease in the oxygen content of blood flowing through the brain
(D) a decrease in the metabolic rate of the surrounding brain tissue
(E) an increase in the pH of the CSF

255. In an acclimatized person at high altitudes, oxygen delivery to the tissues may be adequate at rest because of

(A) an increase in hemoglobin concentration
(B) the presence of an acidosis
(C) a decrease in the number of tissue capillaries
(D) the presence of a normal arterial P_{O_2}
(E) the presence of a lower-than-normal arterial P_{CO_2}

256. Which of the following will increase as a result of stimulating parasympathetic nerves to the bronchial smooth muscle?

(A) Lung compliance
(B) Airway diameter
(C) Elastic work of breathing
(D) Resistive work of breathing
(E) Anatomic dead space

257. During a normal inspiration, more air goes to the alveoli at the base of the lung than to the alveoli at the apex of the lung because

(A) the alveoli at the base of the lung have more surfactant
(B) the alveoli at the base of the lung are more compliant
(C) the alveoli at the base of the lung have higher V/Q ratios
(D) there is a more negative intrapleural pressure at the base of the lung
(E) there is more blood flow to the base of the lung

258. A spirometer can be used to measure directly

(A) functional residual capacity
(B) inspiratory capacity
(C) residual volume
(D) total lung capacity
(E) none of the above

DIRECTIONS: Each numbered question or incomplete statement below is NEGATIVELY phrased. Select the **one best** lettered response.

259. The oxygen required by the respiratory muscles would be increased by all the following EXCEPT

(A) a decrease in lung compliance
(B) a decrease in airway resistance
(C) an increase in the rate of respiration
(D) a decrease in the production of pulmonary surfactant
(E) an increase in tidal volume

260. Functions of alveolar macrophages include all the following EXCEPT

(A) phagocytosis of bacteria
(B) secretion of surfactant
(C) release of lysosomal enzymes into the alveolar space
(D) transport of inhaled particles out of the alveoli
(E) release of leukocyte chemotactic factors

261. Characteristics of blood in the pulmonary circulation include all the following EXCEPT

(A) volume of about 1 L
(B) flow rate of about 5.5 L/min
(C) volume in the capillaries of less than 100 mL
(D) flow rate that increases during exercise
(E) flow that is nonpulsatile

262. All the following are characteristics of the lung EXCEPT

(A) the interstitial colloid oncotic pressure is about 15 mmHg
(B) filtration is continuous along the length of the alveolar capillary
(C) the hydrostatic pressure in the pulmonary capillaries is the same as in the systemic capillaries
(D) filtered H_2O is removed by the lymphatics
(E) the interstitial hydrostatic pressure is subatmospheric

263. In a normal, standing person, all the following will contribute significantly to the existence of the alveolar-arterial (A-a) gradient for O_2 EXCEPT

(A) variations in the V/Q ratios throughout the lungs
(B) a small right-to-left absolute shunt
(C) the nonlinearity of the oxyhemoglobin dissociation curve
(D) the disequilibrium of end-pulmonary capillary P_{O_2} and alveolar P_{O_2}
(E) blood flow from the bronchial circulation

264. Surfactant is accurately described by all the following statements EXCEPT

(A) it is a lipoprotein containing dipalmitoyl lecithin
(B) it is responsible for the hysteresis demonstrated in the pressure-volume curve characteristics of the human lung
(C) it reduces surface tension in the alveoli
(D) it is made in type II cells
(E) it is present in increased amounts in hyaline membrane disease

265. Metabolic functions of the lung include all the following EXCEPT

(A) inactivation of angiotensin II
(B) inactivation of bradykinin
(C) inactivation of prostaglandins
(D) synthesis of prostaglandins
(E) synthesis of surfactant

266. Factors in determining the diffusion capacity of the lung for oxygen $(D_L O_2)$ include all the following EXCEPT

(A) the cardiac output
(B) the oxygen partial pressure gradient from alveolar gas to pulmonary capillary blood
(C) the concentration of hemoglobin in the pulmonary capillary blood
(D) the alveolar surface area
(E) the thickness of the alveolar-capillary membrane

267. Venous admixture is produced by blood from all the following EXCEPT

(A) the thebesian veins
(B) high V/Q areas of the lung
(C) the bronchial veins
(D) right-to-left intracardiac shunts
(E) alveoli with impaired diffusion

268. In a normal person, end-pulmonary capillary blood would reach diffusional equilibrium with the alveolar partial pressure of all the following EXCEPT

(A) oxygen
(B) nitrogen
(C) carbon dioxide
(D) carbon monoxide
(E) nitrous oxide (N_2O)

269. Shift of the CO_2 response curve from curve A to curve B as shown below would be produced by all the following EXCEPT

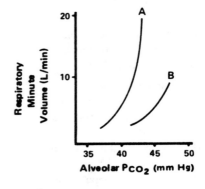

(A) diazepam
(B) barbiturates
(C) morphine
(D) sleep
(E) exercise

270. Hypoxemia ($Pa_{O_2} = 55$ mmHg) has all the following effects EXCEPT

(A) it stimulates carotid body chemoreceptors
(B) it stimulates central chemoreceptors
(C) it stimulates aortic body chemoreceptors
(D) it causes a reflex increase in ventilation
(E) it causes a reflex increase in arterial blood pressure

271. Hyperventilation may be produced by stimulation of all the following receptors EXCEPT

(A) peripheral chemoreceptors
(B) irritant receptors
(C) peripheral pain receptors
(D) pulmonary stretch receptors
(E) J (juxtacapillary) receptors

272. A pulmonary arterial (Swan-Ganz) catheter can be used for all the following EXCEPT

(A) to measure pulmonary artery diastolic pressure
(B) to measure pulmonary artery systolic pressure
(C) to measure pulmonary capillary wedge pressure
(D) to estimate aortic pressure
(E) to estimate left atrial pressure

DIRECTIONS: Each group of questions below consists of lettered headings followed by a set of numbered items. For each numbered item select the **one** lettered heading with which it is **most** closely associated. Each lettered heading may be used **once, more than once, or not at all**.

Questions 273–277

For blood under each of the conditions described below, select the oxyhemoglobin dissociation curve with which it is most likely to be associated. The normal dissociation oxyhemoglobin curve is labeled N.

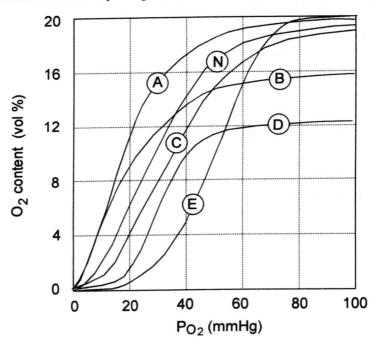

273. Fetal blood

274. Blood stored for 3 weeks

275. Anemic blood

276. Blood from a person who has acclimatized to high altitude

277. Blood exposed to carbon monoxide

Questions 278–279

The tracings below, which represent the maximum flow that can be achieved by a subject during a forced expiration, are called *flow-volume curves*. The thick tracing represents a flow-volume curve from a normal subject. Choose the tracing that was most likely obtained from each of the following persons.

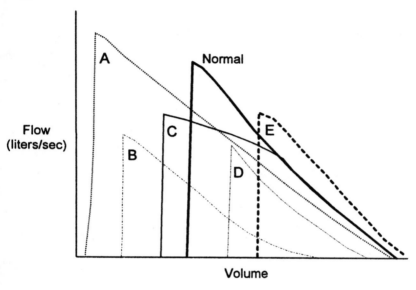

278. A patient with emphysema

279. A patient with a restrictive lung disease

Questions 280–283

For each of the situations described, choose the combination of arterial blood gas changes in the table with which it is most likely to be associated.

	ph	Pa_{CO_2}	Pa_{O_2}
(A)	↑	↑	↑
(B)	↓	↑	↑
(C)	↑	↑	↓
(D)	↓	↓	↑
(E)	↓	↑	↓
(F)	↑	↓	↑
(G)	↑	↓	↓

280. A large intrapulmonary shunt

281. Sudden ascension to a high altitude

282. Metabolic acidosis

283. Respiratory arrest

Respiratory Physiology
Answers

204. The answer is C. *(West, 12/e, pp 579–580.)* The basic respiratory rhythm originates from spontaneous rhythmic discharge of inspiratory neurons located in the respiratory center in the dorsal medulla. This basic rhythm can be modified by many factors, including voluntary control of breathing. In the pons are the apneustic center and the pneumotaxic center (which is located in the nucleus parabrachialis). These modify and regularize the basic respiratory rhythm to produce adequate breathing.

205. The answer is C. *(West, 5/e, pp 103–104.)* During inspiration, the pressure in the alveoli becomes negative and gas is drawn into the lung by the difference in pressure between the alveoli and the atmosphere. At the peak of a normal inspiration, this pressure difference is only a few centimeters of water. At the end of inspiration, the pressure in the alveoli becomes equal to the atmospheric pressure and flow ceases. During expiration, the intraalveolar pressure rises above atmospheric pressure and gas is expelled from the lungs. The intraalveolar pressure again equals atmospheric pressure at the end of expiration.

206. The answer is B. *(West, 5/e, pp 12–14.)* Functional residual capacity (FRC) is the volume of gas in the lung at the end of a normal expiration when the muscles of inspiration and expiration are relaxed. At FRC the elastic forces acting on the lungs are in equilibrium; that is, the tendency of the lungs to collapse is balanced by the tendency of the chest to expand. The volume of gas remaining in the lung at the end of a maximal expiration is the residual volume (RV). RV cannot be measured by spirometry. The vital capacity (VC) is the maximum amount of gas that can be exhaled after a subject inhales maximally. VC, which can be determined from the spirometry tracing, equals 4 L. Since RV equals TLC (6 L) minus VC (4 L), the RV is equal to 2 L. The FRC is 1 L greater than the RV and therefore must be 3 L.

207. The answer is C. *(West, 5/e, pp 148–150.)* The FEV_1 is the amount of gas that can be expelled from the lungs in 1 s during a force expiration from total lung capacity (TLC). Based on the spirometry tracing, FEV_1 equals 3.5 L. The FEV_1 is normally about 85 percent of VC, so the patient has a normal FEV_1. The FEV_1 can be decreased by an obstructive disease such as asthma or emphysema. In a restrictive disease, the FEV_1 is also lower than normal, but the ratio of FEV_1 to VC is normal or slightly higher than normal.

208. The answer is E. *(Berne, 3/e, pp 558–559.)* The inspiratory capacity (IC) is the maximum amount of gas that can be inhaled when the subject starts from functional residual capacity (FRC). In this subject the IC is 3 L. The maximum amount of gas that can be inhaled when the subject starts at the end of a normal inspiration is called the *inspiratory reserve volume (IRV)*. In this subject the IRV equals 2.5 L. The expiratory reserve volume (ERV) is the maximum amount of gas that can be exhaled when the subject starts from FRC. In this subject the ERV equals 1 L.

209. The answer is E. *(Berne, 3/e, pp 555, 560, 609–610. Ganong, 16/e, pp 624–625. West, 5/e, pp 131–132.)* The modified alveolar gas equation

$$PA_{O_2} = PI_{O_2} - \frac{PA_{CO_2}}{R}$$

can be used to calculate the alveolar oxygen tension. The inspired oxygen tension is 21 percent of dry air pressure, which is atmospheric pressure minus water vapor pressure ($P_{ATM} - P_{H_2O}$). The water vapor pressure is assumed to be 47 mmHg because the inspired gas is at body temperature and 100 percent saturated with water. R, the respiratory exchange ratio, is assumed to be 0.8. This value varies with the concentration of oxygen in the inspired gas and diet. When 100% oxygen is breathed or when the diet is exclusively carbohydrates, R equals 1.0. Since the atmospheric pressure is 400 mmHg and his PA_{CO_2} is 30 mmHg, his PA_{O_2} is

$$0.21 \cdot (400 - 47) - 30 \div 0.8 = 37 \text{ mmHg.}$$

210. The answer is C. *(West, 5/e, pp 12–13, 150.)* After performing a forced vital capacity test, the amount of gas remaining in the lung is the residual volume (RV). Since the RV remains in the lung, it cannot be measured by spirometry. Because the FRC and TLC are composed, in part, by the RV, their values cannot be determined by spirometry either. However, their values can be determined by a gas dilution technique in which a known amount of helium (A_{He}) is equilibrated with a volume of gas. By measuring the concentration of helium (C_{He}) in a sample of gas and knowing the total amount of helium present, the volume of gas (V) can be determined, since $V = A_{He}/C_{He}$. In practice, the helium is added to the lung by having the patient breathe into a spirometer containing a known amount of gas (V_S) with a known concentration of helium (C_{HeS}). A_{He} is then $V_S \bullet C_{HeS}$, V is the sum of the lung volume being measured (V_L) and the spirometry volume (V_S), and $C_{He\,(L+S)}$ is the concentration of helium in the spirometer after equilibration is achieved.

$$V_L + V_S = \frac{V_S \bullet C_{HeS}}{C_{HeL}}$$

In this case, the subject is connected to the spirometer after she has performed a maximum expiration, so the lung volume measured by the gas dilution technique is the residual volume. Substituting in the above equation yields an RV of

$$12\,L \bullet (0.1 \div 0.085) - 12\,L = 2.1\,L.$$

Since her vital capacity is 5 L, her TLC is 7 L.

211. The answer is A. *(Berne, 3/e, pp 568–569.)* Normal lung volumes depend on posture because the position of the body influences the balance of forces that determine these volumes. For example, when a person lies down, the abdominal contents push against the diaphragm, making the resting lung volume (the FRC) smaller. The other lung volumes may change as well, but because their values are primarily determined by muscular effort, they will normally not change very much. If the person is very obese, then the stomach contents may have a large effect on the other lung volumes.

212–213. The answers are 212-B, 213-D. *(Berne, 3/e, pp 559–560. West, 5/e, pp 14–17.)* Alveolar ventilation (VA) is the amount of gas per minute that enters the respiratory exchange areas of the lung and is equal to the minute ventilation (V_{MIN}) minus the dead space ventilation (V_D):

$$VA = V_{min} - V_D$$
$$VA = (18 \bullet 350) - (18 \bullet 100) = 4500\,mL = 4.5\,L$$

Because all the CO_2 eliminated (V_{CO_2}) enters the alveolar gas, the concentration of CO_2 in the alveoli (FA_{CO_2}) is equal to $\dot{V}_{CO_2}/VA$. Assuming that the amount of CO_2 produced each minute does not change with changes in ventilation, then

$$\dot{V}_{CO_2} = FA'_{CO_2} \bullet \dot{V}A' = FA''_{CO_2} \bullet \dot{V}A''$$

or since PA_{CO_2} is proportional to FA_{CO_2}

$$PA'_{CO_2} \bullet \dot{V}A' = PA''_{CO_2} \bullet \dot{V}A''$$

If her tidal volume increases from 350 mL to 425 mL, then her alveolar ventilation becomes $18 \cdot (425 - 100)$, or 5850 mL/min, and her $V_{A_{CO_2}}$ decreases from a normal value of 40 mmHg to

$$PA_{CO_2} = \frac{40 \cdot 4500}{5850} = 30.8 \text{ mmHg}$$

214–215. The answers are 214-B, 215-C. *(Berne, 3/e, pp 572–573. West, 5/e, pp 107–110.)* The equal pressure point is the point at which the pressure inside the airways equals the intrapleural pressure. If the equal pressure point occurs where the bronchioles can collapse, the airway will narrow and the maximum expiratory flow rate will be limited. The intraairway pressure at the beginning of the airways (closest to the alveoli) equals the sum of the recoil pressure (exerted by the alveoli) and the intrapleural pressure (produced by the muscles of expiration). Therefore, the intraairway pressure at the alveoli equals 40 cmH$_2$O (10 cmH$_2$O + 30 cmH$_2$O). Assuming that the intraairway pressure is zero at the mouth and drops linearly from the alveoli to the mouth, the intraairway pressure will be 30 cmH$_2$O one-fourth of the way down the airway, 20 cmH$_2$O one-half of the way down the airway, and 10 cmH$_2$O three-fourths of the way down the airway. Since the intrapleural pressure is 30 cmH$_2$O, the equal pressure point will be approximately one-fourth of the way down the airway (point B).

The equal pressure point moves further away from the lungs if the recoil force is increased and moves closer to the lungs when the intrapleural pressure is increased. Increasing the lung volume expands the alveoli and makes their recoil force greater. This moves the equal pressure point toward the mouth. If airway resistance increases, for example by increasing airway smooth muscle tone, then a greater expiratory effort and consequently a greater intrapleural pressure will be necessary to expel the gas from the lungs.

216. The answer is D. *(West, 5/e, pp 148–151.)* Obstructive lung disease is characterized by an increased resistance to airflow, which makes it more difficult to expel gas from the lung during expiration. As a result, the amount of gas in the lung at the end of each expiration, the functional residual capacity (FRC), increases. The increased airway resistance limits the rate at which gas can be expired, and so maximum breathing capacity, FEV$_1$, and breathing frequency all decrease. Vital capacity usually decreases because of gas trapping. In restrictive disease, the decreased lung compliance causes vital capacity (VC) and FRC to decrease. The decreased compliance also reduces the amount of air that can be inhaled with each breath, so maximum breathing capacity and FEV$_1$ decrease. At the same time, breathing frequency has to increase to compensate for the decreased tidal volume.

217. The answer is A. *(Berne, 3/e, pp 572–573.)* During the early stages of an asthmatic attack, the increased airway resistance makes it difficult to inhale and exhale rapidly, and therefore each breath is slower and deeper. However, the accompanying dyspnea usually increases alveolar ventilation, and as a result PA_{CO_2} decreases. Arterial oxygen tension usually decreases, despite normal alveolar oxygen levels, because of the increased V/Q mismatch that accompanies asthma. This hypoxia may also cause alveolar ventilation to increase. The equal pressure point moves toward the lung because of the increased respiratory effort. Acute asthmatic attacks do not produce any direct change in lung compliance. However, air trapping will cause functional residual capacity (FRC) to increase, and the larger lung volumes will lead to a decrease in lung compliance.

218. The answer is C. *(West, 5/e, pp 64–67.)* $\dot{V}/\dot{Q}$ mismatches will cause arterial oxygen levels (Pa_{O_2}) to decrease. Arterial carbon dioxide levels (Pa_{CO_2}) tend to remain normal, however, because the central chemoreceptors increase ventilation to keep Pa_{CO_2} at 40 mmHg. The hypoxia may lead to a lactic acidosis that decreases pH and increases the anion gap. The increased ventilation will increase alveolar oxygen tension (PA_{O_2}) slightly, which, coupled with the decreased PA_{O_2}, will lead to an increased A-a gradient for oxygen (PA_{O_2} - Pa_{O_2}).

219. The answer is A. *(West, 5/e, pp 61–64.)* The alveoli at the apex of the lung are larger than those at the base so their compliance is less. Because of the reduced compliance, less inspired gas goes to the apex than to the base. Also, because the apex is above the heart, less blood flows through the apex than through the base. However, the reduction in air flow is less than the reduction in blood flow, so that the $\dot{V}/\dot{Q}$ ratio at the top of the lung is greater than it is at the bottom. The increased $\dot{V}/\dot{Q}$ ratio at the apex makes PA_{CO_2} lower and PA_{O_2} higher at the apex than they are at the base.

220. The answer is D. *(West, 5/e, pp 126–127.)* Under normal conditions, alveolar ventilation is controlled by the central chemoreceptors, which increase ventilation in response to an increase in Pa_{CO_2} or a decrease in pH. Prolonged hypoxemia, as often occurs in patients with chronic respiratory disease, depresses the central chemoreceptors and prevents them from stimulating respiration. When this happens, the peripheral chemoreceptors, which are stimulated by low arterial oxygen tension, provide the only drive to ventilation. Providing oxygen under these conditions produces apnea by removing the peripheral chemoreceptor drive at the same time that the central chemoreceptors are depressed.

221. The answer is D. *(West, 5/e, p 10.)* The lung has a variety of mechanisms to remove particulate matter from the inspired gas. Large particles become deposited in the mucus layer that lies within the bronchi. The mucus is swept up and out of the bronchioles by the ciliated epithelial cells that line the bronchioles. Smaller particles remain suspended in the inspired gas and reach the alveoli. Alveolar macrophages remove these particles by phagocytosis. The macrophages are usually removed from the lung through the lymphatic or blood circulation. Cigarette smoking can prevent cilia from beating, reduce macrophage migration, and thus impair the ability of the lungs to remove potentially harmful particles inhaled from the atmosphere.

222. The answer is E. *(Ganong, 16/e, pp 623–630.)* Low arterial oxygen tension (mmHg) results from hypoventilation, decreased oxygen in the inspired air, or $\dot{V}/\dot{Q}$ abnormalities. Low oxygen content (mL of O_2 per 100 mL of blood) results from low oxygen tension, anemia (reduced numbers of red blood cells or reduced hemoglobin), or reduced affinity of hemoglobin for oxygen. Respiratory acidosis is caused by a decrease in alveolar ventilation, which leads to an increase in P_{CO_2} and a decrease in P_{O_2} and O_2 content. Fever may decrease the affinity of hemoglobin for oxygen and thus reduce oxygen content, but will not directly affect oxygen tension. In fact, oxygen tension may increase because fever increases ventilation. Carbon monoxide reduces the affinity of Hb for O_2 but has no direct effect on P_{O_2}.

223. The answer is D. *(Berne, 3/e, pp 596–598.)* CO_2 is transported in arterial blood in three forms: as physically dissolved CO_2 (about 5 percent), in combination with the amino groups of hemoglobin as carbaminohemoglobin (about 5 percent), and as bicarbonate ion HCO_3^- (about 90 percent). The amount of CO_2 actually carried as carbonic acid (H_2CO_3) is negligible. Carboxyhemoglobin refers to the combination of carbon monoxide (CO) and hemoglobin.

224. The answer is B. *(West, 12/e, pp 518–520.)* In humans, the airway begins with the trachea and major bronchi and terminates in the alveolar sacs. The trachea and bronchi (A in the diagram accompanying the question) are lined by ciliated columnar epithelium with numerous mucous glands that provide lubrication and cleansing action. The distal airway includes the terminal bronchiole (B), respiratory bronchiole (C), alveolar duct (D), and alveolar sacs (E). The surface distal to the terminal bronchiole is covered by a thin epithelial lining that is separated from the interstitium and capillary wall by a thin basement membrane. This "respiratory membrane" has an overall thickness ranging from 0.2 to 0.5 μ. It is across this surface that CO_2 and O_2 exchange occurs by passive diffusion. In adults, the total surface area across which this exchange occurs is approximately 70 m². Because total pulmonary capillary blood volume is approximately 100 mL, gas exchange is rapid.

225. The answer is C. *(West, 12/e, p 521.)* According to Dalton's law of partial pressures, each component in a gas mixture exerts a pressure proportional to its concentration in the mixture, and the sum of the pressures of the components is equal to the total pressure of the gas. In air at 4 atmospheres (4 × 760 mmHg) the partial pressure of oxygen would be 0.21 × 4 × 760 = 640 mmHg. Long-term exposure to such an elevated P_{O_2} can have harmful effects on both pulmonary and neural function.

226. The answer is C. *(West, 12/e, pp 524–525.)* Alveolar ventilation is found as follows:

$$(\text{Tidal volume} - \text{dead space volume}) \times \text{frequency}$$

In the example provided in the question, the patient's and the machine's dead spaces must be added to determine the total dead space in each breath (of 1 L). Thus, alveolar ventilation = (1000 mL − 200 mL − 50 mL) × 10/min = 7.5 L/min.

227. The answer is D. *(West, 12/e, pp 523–527.)* Changes in tidal volume (TV) have a greater effect on alveolar ventilation ($\dot{V}_A$) than do equivalent changes in respiratory rate (RR) because of the contribution of the dead space. This relationship can be seen from the expression

$$\dot{V}_A = RR\,(TV - \text{dead space})$$

Assuming, for example, that TV = 500 mL, RR = 12/min, and dead space = 150 mL,

$$\dot{V}_A = 12\,(500 - 150) = 4200 \text{ mL/min}$$

If TV is doubled and RR halved,

$$TV \times 2 = 1000 \text{ mL}$$
$$RR \div 2 = 6/\text{min}$$
$$\text{and } \dot{V}_A = 6\,(1000 - 150) = 5100 \text{ mL/min}$$

But if TV is halved and RR doubled,

$$TV \div 2 = 250 \text{ mL}$$
$$RR \times 2 = 24/\text{min}$$
$$\dot{V}_A = 24 \ (250 - 150) = 2400 \text{ mL/min}$$

228. The answer is A. *(Guyton, 8/e, pp 424–426.)* The anatomic dead space, which includes the trachea, bronchi, and bronchioles, is filled with fresh room air at the end of an inspiration and with end-expired, or alveolar, gas at the end of an expiration. Room air contains very little CO_2 (0.03 percent), whereas alveolar air contains considerably more CO_2 (about 5.5 percent) as a result of gas exchange in the lungs. The P_{CO_2} of alveolar air does fluctuate to some extent with each breath because it is diluted with fresh air during inspiration. The P_{CO_2} of the blood in the pulmonary veins is in equilibrium with that in the alveoli.

229. The answer is C. *(West, 12/e, pp 580–582, 583–585.)* The central chemoreceptors located on or near the ventral surface of the medulla cause an increase in ventilation in response to an increase in Pa_{CO_2} and to a lesser extent to a decrease in arterial pH because the blood-brain barrier is relatively impermeable to hydrogen ions. The peripheral chemoreceptors in the carotid bodies cause an increase in ventilation in response to an increase in Pa_{CO_2}, a decrease in arterial pH, and a decrease in Pa_{O_2}. Neither the central chemoreceptors nor the carotid bodies are stimulated by a decrease in arterial blood pressure or O_2 content.

230. The answer is B. *(Ganong, 16/e, pp 611–613.)* Transection of the brainstem above the pons would prevent any voluntary changes in ventilation by cutting the pathways from the higher centers. Breathing would continue because the pontine-medullary centers that control rhythmic ventilation would be intact. Inputs to the brainstem from the central and peripheral chemoreceptors that stimulate ventilation and from lung stretch receptors that inhibit inspiration (Hering-Breuer reflex) would also be intact and these reflexes would be maintained.

231–232. The answers are 231-B, 232-C. *(West, 12/e, pp 569–570.)* During inspiration (curve ABC) the respiratory muscles pull the chest wall out and diaphragm down and intrapleural pressure (P_{IP}) becomes more negative. The muscles must overcome the elastic recoil forces of the lungs and the resistance of the airways to airflow. The P_{IP} necessary to overcome the elastic forces of the lung is depicted by dashed line AC. The P_{IP} necessary to overcome the airway resistance is the difference between dashed line AC and curve ABC. The maximum airflow occurs at point B, where the difference between the two is the greatest. Lung volume is the greatest at point C, where P_{IP} is the most negative.

233. The answer is B. *(Berne, 3/e, p 555. West, 12/e, p 521.)* Water vapor pressure is independent of the barometric pressure and depends only on the temperature of a gas and the percentage of saturation. By the time inspired gas reaches the alveoli it is at body temperature (37°C) and fully saturated with water. Water vapor pressure of saturated gas at 37°C is 47 mmHg.

234. The answer is C. *(West, 12/e, pp 561–566.)* Because of the inherent elasticity of the lung, the alveoli tend to collapse during expiration. This tendency is explained by Laplace's law, which relates the radius (R) and surface tension (T) of an elastic bubble to the pressure (P) required to distend it, as follows: $P = 2T \div R$. If T were constant, the pressure required to distend alveoli would increase markedly during expiration as the radius decreased. This does not occur in normal lungs because the unique properties of surfactant result in reduced surface tension as the alveolar lining is compressed with the decrease in the alveolar radius during expiration. Thus, surfactant prevents alveolar collapse at end-expiratory intraalveolar pressures that otherwise would lead to atelectasis. A deficiency of surfactant would therefore increase surface tension, tending to collapse the lungs and decrease FRC. It would be more difficult to expand the lungs. Lung compliance would decrease, and thus a greater change in intrapleural pressure and greater work to maintain ventilation would be required.

235–236. The answers are 235-D, 236-A. *(West, 12/e, pp 575–576.)* In the diagram accompanying the question, zones I through IV represent gas from different topographical areas of the lung. Zone I represents dead space, zone II is a mixture of dead space and alveolar gas, and zone III represents pure alveolar gas. At point D the tracer content of expired gas increases. That point represents the closing volume, which is the lung volume at which airways in the lower parts of the lung close off because the transmural pressure gradient is lower owing to the effects of gravity. The gas in the apices (zone IV) is richer in the tracer gas because the alveoli in that portion of the lung receive more gas during the early part of inspiration. The closing volume represents approximately 10 percent of vital capacity and increases with age, as does residual volume.

237. The answer is B. *(West, 12/e, pp 18, 19.)* The volume of the physiologic dead space (V_D) can be calculated using the Bohr equation:

$$V_D = \left(\frac{FA_{CO_2} - FE_{CO_2}}{FA_{CO_2}} \right) V_T$$

V_T is tidal volume, FA_{CO_2} is the fraction of CO_2 in alveolar gas, and FE_{CO_2} is the fraction of CO_2 in mixed expired gas. FA_{CO_2} can be approximated using the F_{CO_2} from a sample of end-expiratory gas or by sampling Pa_{CO_2}. In normal lungs, physiologic dead space equals anatomic dead space. In diseased lungs, physiologic dead space often exceeds anatomic dead space because of abnormalities of ventilation and blood flow.

238. The answer is D. *(West, 12/e, pp 546–548, 559.)* In patients, it is useful to calculate the alveolar oxygen tension (PA_{O_2}) in order to assess the alveolar-arterial oxygen gradient. PA_{O_2} can be calculated using the alveolar gas equation:

$$PA_{O_2} = PI_{O_2} - PA_{CO_2}\left(FI_{O_2} + \frac{1 - FI_{O_2}}{R}\right)$$

This equation can be greatly simplified without sacrificing a great deal of accuracy. The modified alveolar gas equation is

$$PA_{O_2} = PI_{O_2} - \frac{PA_{CO_2}}{R}$$

PA_{CO_2} is equivalent to Pa_{CO_2}. R is the respiratory exchange ratio ($\dot{V}CO_2/\dot{V}O_2$), which depends on the diet and is normally 0.8. PI_{O_2} equals the fraction of oxygen in room air (0.21) times the barometric pressure at sea level (760 mmHg) minus the water vapor pressure (47 mmHg) of saturated tracheal gas at body temperature (37°C).

$$PA_{O_2} = 0.21\,(760\text{ mmHg} - 47\text{ mmHg}) - \frac{48\text{ mmHg}}{0.8}$$
$$= 150\text{ mmHg} - 60\text{ mmHg}$$
$$= 90\text{ mmHg}$$

239. The answer is B. *(West, 12/e, pp 554–558.)* Under normal conditions the V/Q ratio in both lungs is the same, so that mixed alveolar gas in the trachea has the same P_{O_2} and P_{CO_2} as arterial blood ($P_{O_2} = 100$ mmHg, $P_{CO_2} = 40$ mmHg). Immediately following complete occlusion of one pulmonary artery, however, equal ventilation of both lungs continues, but all blood flow is directed to one lung. Equal volumes of gas will continue to mix in the trachea, but the gas from the occluded lung, which now represents alveolar dead space, will be unchanged from room air ($P_{O_2} = 150$ mmHg, $P_{CO_2} = 0.3$ mmHg); and gas from the functioning lung will still be normal ($P_{O_2} = 100$ mmHg,

$P_{CO_2} = 40$ mmHg). Since equal volumes of gas mix, P_{O_2} in the trachea will be $(150 + 100) \div 2$, or 125 mmHg, and P_{CO_2} will be $(40 + 0.3) \div 2$, or 20 mmHg. Such values could occur in normal lungs following hyperventilation but would be accompanied by changes in arterial P_{CO_2}.

240. The answer is E. *(Ganong, 16/e, pp 594–595.)* Lecithin (phosphatidylcholine) and sphingomyelin are choline phospholipids found in a variety of tissues. Lecithin is a major component of surfactant and its synthesis increases as the fetus matures and the lungs are prepared for expansion. Surfactant, a lipoprotein mixture, prevents alveolar collapse by permitting the surface tension of the alveolar lining to vary during inspiration and expiration. Thus, measurement of the lecithin-sphingomyelin (L-S) ratio in amniotic fluid provides an index of fetal lung maturity.

241. The answer is C. *(Berne, 3/e, pp 558–559.)* The lungs tend to recoil inward, whereas the chest wall tends to recoil outward. When the respiratory muscles are all relaxed, these two opposing forces are balanced. The volume of gas in the lungs at this point is the relaxation volume, or functional residual capacity (FRC).

242. The answer is C. *(Berne 3/e, pp 559–560, 602–603, 606–607. West, 12/e, pp 546–548, 558.)* A high arterial P_{CO_2} is most likely caused by depressed medullary respiratory centers. Depression of these centers decreases alveolar ventilation and results in hypoventilation with an increased Pa_{CO_2} and decreased Pa_{O_2}. This depression can be caused by drugs such as barbiturates or narcotics. Slight depression also occurs during sleep. If metabolic activity increases, as during mild exercise, alveolar ventilation increases in parallel and Pa_{CO_2} does not change. Retention of CO_2 could result from alveolar capillary block, but it would have to be extremely severe because CO_2 is so soluble in tissue.

243. The answer is E. *(West, 12/e, pp 568–572.)* Although it may seem paradoxical, about 80 percent of the total resistance to airflow occurs in the large- and medium-sized airways. Turbulent flow, which increases the pressure necessary to cause gas to flow, is more likely to occur in larger airways. In patients, an increased resistance to airflow usually indicates the presence of disease of the large airways.

244. The answer is A. *(West, 12/e, pp 530–532.)* Pulmonary vascular resistance changes as lung volume changes. At TLC, expansion of the alveoli increases the pulmonary vascular resistance by compressing the alveolar capillaries. At RV, there is compression of the extraalveolar vessels, which increases the pulmonary vascular resistance. At FRC, the compression by either mechanism is minimal. Pulmonary vascular resistance decreases as left atrial pressure increases, as cardiac output increases, or as pulmonary artery pressure increases because of recruitment and distension of pulmonary capillaries.

245. The answer is D. *(Ganong, 16/e, pp 484, 568–569. West, 12/e, pp 898–900.)* Because fetal hemoglobin (hemoglobin F) is chemically different from adult hemoglobin in that is has two α and two γ chains instead of two α and two β chains, it has a greater affinity for oxygen. This is advantageous in the placental exchange of O_2 from maternal blood (Pa_{O_2} = 100 mmHg) to fetal blood (Pa_{O_2} = 25 mmHg). Pa_{CO_2} is about 2 to 3 mmHg higher in the fetus than in the mother. $[H^+]a$ is about the same in both. Pulmonary vascular resistance is high in the fetus, shunting blood away from the lungs. It decreases at birth and remains low.

246. The answer is C. *(West, 12/e, pp 89–91.)* Expiration is normally a passive process that does not require the involvement of any muscles. In a forced expiration the internal intercostal muscles contract, pulling the rib cage downward. The abdominal muscles also contract, which increases intraabdominal pressure and pulls the rib cage downward and inward. The diaphragm and external intercostal muscles contract during inspiration. The scalene and sternocleidomastoid muscles, which assist in expanding the chest wall in inspiration, are important accessory muscles of respiration.

247. The answer is D. *(Berne, 3/e, pp 607–608. Ganong, 16/e, pp 620–622.)* During moderate aerobic exercise, oxygen consumption and CO_2 production increase, but alveolar ventilation increases in parallel. Thus, Pa_{O_2} and Pa_{CO_2} do not change. Arterial pH does not decrease and blood lactate concentration does not increase during moderate aerobic exercise, but arterial pH does decrease and blood lactate concentration does increase during anaerobic exercise because of increased production of lactic acid.

248. The answer is E. *(Ganong, 16/e, pp 613–616.)* The reduction in functional hemoglobin that occurs in anemia, methemoglobinemia, or carboxyhemoglobinemia lessens the total oxygen *content* (dissolved O_2 + HbO_2) in the blood but not the oxygen *tension* (P_{O_2}). Because the chemoreceptors of the carotid body are sensitive to the P_{O_2} of arterial blood and blood flow to the carotid body is normally very high, under conditions in which dissolved oxygen and P_{O_2} are normal the amount of O_2 delivered per unit time is sufficient to prevent activation of the chemoreceptors and no hyperpnea ensues. Central chemoreceptors are stimulated by decreases in the pH of brain extracellular fluid. They do not respond to changes in P_{O_2}.

249. The answer is B. *(West, 12/e, pp 535–536.)* The forces tending to remove fluid from the alveoli are the negative interstitial fluid pressure and the osmotic pressure exerted at the alveolar membrane by ions and crystalloid molecules in the interstitial fluid. Fluid movement into pulmonary *capillaries*, however, is a function of plasma *oncotic* pressure. The pulmonary capillaries are actually leakier than those in the systemic circulation; i.e., they have a higher hydraulic conductivity. Alveolar phagocytes do not take up significant amounts of water, and very little water from the alveoli goes into inspired air because the air is well humidified by the upper airways. Surfactant lowers the surface tension in the alveoli but does not affect fluid movement.

250. The answer is C. *(Berne, 3/e, pp 596–598. West, 5/e, pp 76–79.)* In the tissues, CO_2 diffuses into the blood down its concentration gradient. CO_2 enters the red cells where carbonic anhydrase accelerates its hydration reaction.

$$CO_2 + H_2O \overset{CA}{\rightleftharpoons} H_2CO_3 \rightleftharpoons H^+ + HCO_3^-$$

Thus, the concentration of H^+ and HCO_3^- in the red cell rise. Most of the H^+ is buffered by hemoglobin, but the new HCO_3^- ion constitutes a new osmotic particle in the red cell and the red cell swells. Most of the HCO_3^- exchanges for Cl^- across the red cell membrane, which increases the amount of the chloride in the red cell. The increased P_{CO_2} and concentration of H^+ cause a decrease in the affinity of hemoglobin for O_2.

251. The answer is D. *(Berne, 3/e, pp 591–594.)* The percentage of hemoglobin saturated with oxygen depends on the level of P_{O_2} in the blood and on other factors that affect the position of the oxyhemoglobin dissociation curve. Factors that shift the curve to the left, such as a decrease in P_{CO_2}, an increase in pH, or a decrease in temperature, would increase the percentage of hemoglobin saturated with oxygen as would an increase in P_{O_2} provided that the percentage of saturation was not already at 100 percent. At a given P_{O_2}, increasing the concentration of hemoglobin would not affect the percentage of saturation but would increase the oxygen content of blood.

252. The answer is A. *(West, 12/e, pp 588–592.)* At high altitude, the barometric pressure is reduced, resulting in a decrease in $P_{I_{O_2}}$, which decreases both alveolar and arterial P_{O_2}. If Pa_{O_2} is less than 60 mmHg, the carotid bodies are stimulated and cause hyperventilation, which increases alveolar ventilation and decreases Pa_{CO_2} with a resultant respiratory alkalosis. During acclimatization Pa_{O_2} remains low, ventilation remains high, and therefore Pa_{CO_2} remains low. The kidneys act to lower plasma bicarbonate and return arterial pH toward normal. The oxygen content of arterial blood increases owing to an increase in hematocrit stimulated by the increased production of erythropoietin in the kidney.

253. The answer is B. *(West, 12/e, pp 562–566.)* Pulmonary compliance, defined as the ratio of change of lung volume to the change in pressure required to inflate the lung ($\Delta V/\Delta P$), is an index of lung distensibility. It decreases in patients with pulmonary edema and interstitial fibrosis and increases in patients with emphysema and in persons of advancing years. The stiffer the lung, the lower the pulmonary compliance. Surfactant lowers the surface tension in the alveoli and makes the lung more distensible.

254. The answer is A. *(Berne, 3/e, pp 602–603.)* The central chemoreceptors are located at or near the ventral surface of the medulla. They are stimulated to increase ventilation by a decrease in the pH of their extracellular fluid (ECF). The pH of this ECF is affected by the P_{CO_2} of the blood supply to the medullary chemoreceptor area as well as by the CO_2 and lactic acid production of the surrounding brain tissue. The central chemoreceptors are not stimulated by decreases in Pa_{O_2} or blood oxygen content but rather can be depressed by long-term or severe decreases in oxygen supply.

255. The answer is A. *(Ganong, 16/e, pp 623–626. West, 12/e, pp 538–540, 588–592.)* At a high altitude, arterial P_{O_2} is low because of the low barometric pressure. Ventilation increases owing to stimulation of the carotid body chemoreceptors, and Pa_{O_2} increases somewhat, although it does not return to a normal, sea-level value. With this hyperventilation, Pa_{CO_2} decreases, resulting in a respiratory alkalosis that may become fully compensated with time via renal mechanisms. A lower-than-normal Pa_{CO_2} would shift the oxyhemoglobin dissociation curve to the left, thereby increasing the affinity of hemoglobin for oxygen. Chronic hypoxia at high altitudes or in disease states stimulates the increased release of erythropoietin from the kidneys, which increases the hematocrit and thereby increases the hemoglobin concentration of the blood. Thus at the same lowered Pa_{O_2}, the oxygen content of blood and oxygen delivery to tissues increase. Chronic hypoxia also stimulates increased capillary growth in tissues.

256. The answer is D. *(Berne, 3/e, pp 570–573. West, 12/e, pp 568–572.)* The tone of bronchial smooth muscle is under autonomic control. Stimulation of sympathetic nerves causes bronchodilation, whereas parasympathetic stimulation via the vagus nerve causes bronchoconstriction. Bronchoconstriction reduces the radius of the airways and thereby decreases anatomic dead space and increases airway resistance, which consequently increases the resistive work of breathing. Bronchoconstriction has no significant effect on the elastic properties of the lung.

257. The answer is B. *(West, 12/e, pp 533–534, 554–557, 574–575.)* There is a negative, or subatmospheric, intrapleural pressure (P_{IP}) between the lungs and the chest wall due to the tendency of the chest wall to pull outward and the tendency of the lungs to collapse. Because the lungs are essentially "hanging" in the chest, the force of gravity on the lungs causes the P_{IP} to be more negative at the top of the lung. This also causes the alveoli at the apex (top) of the lung to be larger than those at the base (bottom) of the lung. Larger alveoli are already more inflated and are less compliant than smaller alveoli. During inspiration, when all alveoli are subjected to essentially the same alveolar pressure, more air will go to the more compliant alveoli. Because of the effect of gravity on blood, more blood flow will go to the base of the lung. This does not appreciably affect lung compliance. Ventilation is about three times greater at the base of the lung, but flow is about ten times greater at the base than at the apex of the lung. Therefore, the V/Q ratio is lower at the base than at the apex in a normal lung.

258. The answer is B. *(West, 12/e, pp 522–524.)* A spirometer is an instrument that records the volume of air moved into and out of the lungs during respiration and thus would measure all lung volumes included in maximal inspiration or expiration. Residual volume, which is the volume of gas in the lungs after maximal expiration; functional residual capacity, which is residual volume plus expiratory reserve volume; and total lung capacity, which is the total volume of gas in the lungs after maximal inspiration, cannot be measured directly by a spirometer. They can be measured using a spirometer by gas dilution techniques or by body plethysmography.

259. The answer is B. *(West, 12/e, pp 577–578.)* Respiratory muscles consume oxygen in proportion to the work of breathing, which can be divided into resistance work and compliance, or elastic, work. Resistance work includes work to overcome tissue as well as airway resistance. A decrease in the amount of pulmonary surfactant would decrease lung compliance and increase the elastic work of breathing. An increase in respiratory rate would increase both types of the work of breathing.

260. The answer is B. *(Ganong, 16/e, pp 602–603. West, 12/e, pp 345–346.)* Alveolar macrophages are cells that migrate over the alveolar epithelial surface within the surfactant layer. They are phagocytic cells and ingest inhaled bacteria and particulate matter. This phagocytic activity is often associated with release of leukocyte chemotactic factors and lysosomal enzymes into the extracellular space, which can result in damage to normal tissue by eliciting the inflammatory reaction. Undigested particulate matter is transported out of alveoli by either being carried up the bronchial tree by ciliary action or by circulation through interstitial lymphatic channels. Though macrophages often contain ingested surfactant material, they have not been shown to synthesize surfactant, a product of alveolar type II epithelial cells.

261. The answer is E. *(Ganong, 16/e, pp 599–602.)* The rate of pulmonary blood flow, or the amount of blood entering the lungs per minute, equals the cardiac output. Normally, the lung contains about 1 L of blood, or one-fifth of the total blood volume. Of this, less than 100 mL are contained in capillaries, where most gas exchange occurs. A red blood cell traverses the pulmonary capillaries in about 0.75 s when the body is at rest. During exercise, this time interval may fall to 0.3 s or less, and the rate of pulmonary blood flow may increase to 40 L/min. Blood flow in the pulmonary capillaries is pulsatile.

262. The answer is C. *(West, 5/e, pp 45–47.)* The pulmonary circulation is a low-pressure system. Thus the hydrostatic pressure in the pulmonary capillaries is about 10 mmHg and is less than in the systemic capillaries. It is greater at the base of the lung than at the apex because of increased hydrostatic pressure at the base. The colloid osmotic pressure in the pulmonary capillary is about 25 mmHg and that in the interstitial space is estimated to be about 15 mmHg. The interstitial hydrostatic pressure is estimated to be slightly negative. Thus the balance of these Starling forces favors continuous filtration out of the capillaries into the interstitial space. This continuous flow of fluid is removed by the very efficient lymphatic system in the lungs.

263. The answer is D. *(West, 5/e, pp 52–59.)* In a normal person there is an A-a gradient for O_2 of about 4 to 10 mmHg. The V/Q ratios at the apices of the lungs are greater than at the bases of the lungs; this results in end-pulmonary capillary blood coming from the apices with higher P_{O_2} and from the bases with lower P_{O_2} than normal. The P_{O_2} of the mixed blood from these areas must be determined by the average of their O_2 contents. Because of the nonlinearity of the oxyhemoglobin dissociation curve, the resultant Pa_{O_2} is not the average of the end-pulmonary capillary P_{O_2} values. In addition, about 2 to 5 percent of the blood returning to the left heart—i.e., blood from the bronchial veins and from the thebesian veins draining the left ventricle—is venous blood that has not been oxygenated and constitutes a right-to-left absolute shunt. Normally levels of alveolar and end-pulmonary capillary blood P_{O_2} do come into equilibrium. If they do not, as in some disease states, this alveolar-capillary block would contribute to the A-a gradient for O_2.

264. The answer is E. *(West, 12/e, pp 564–566.)* Surfactant is a lipoprotein mixture rich in dipalmitoyl lecithin, which is made by type II pneumonocytes lining the alveoli. It acts to diminish surface tension when alveolar volume decreases so that the pressure required to maintain the smaller alveolar volume is decreased, thus averting alveolar collapse to zero pressure. Because reexpansion requires sufficient pressure to overcome both surface tension and tissue elasticity, the pressure-volume curves for inflation and deflation do not coincide, and hysteresis results. Hyaline membrane disease (respiratory distress syndrome) results from a deficiency of surfactant and is accompanied by atelectasis.

265. The answer is A. *(West, 12/e, pp 536–537.)* The lung has many metabolic functions, including synthesis of surfactant and prostaglandins and withdrawal of prostaglandins and bradykinin from the circulation. Other metabolic functions include activation of angiotensin I to angiotensin II, release of histamine, and inactivation of serotonin. Prostaglandins E and F both are synthesized and removed from the circulation by the lungs.

266. The answer is B. *(Guyton, 8/e, pp 426–430. West, 5/e, pp 26–28.)* The diffusing capacity of the lung for oxygen (D_LO_2) is the amount of oxygen that crosses the alveolar-capillary membranes per minute per millimeter of mercury of partial pressure difference between the alveolar gas and the pulmonary capillary blood. A normal resting value is about 25 mL/min/mmHg. D_LO_2 depends on the area available for gas exchange, which includes the number of open capillaries in the lung and the thickness of the alveolar-capillary membrane. When cardiac output increases (e.g., during exercise), D_LO_2 increases because more pulmonary capillaries open up. D_LO_2 also depends on the amount of hemoglobin present to take up oxygen in the pulmonary capillary blood.

267. The answer is B. *(West, 12/e, pp 553–556.)* Venous admixture is the addition of blood with a lower P_{O_2} to oxygenated blood returning to the left side of the heart. In a normal person, this lowers the arterial P_{O_2} by about 5 mmHg. This blood includes flow from the thebesian veins, which drain the myocardium of the left ventricle; from the bronchial veins, which drain the walls of the airways; from areas of the lung with lower-than-normal V/Q ratios; and from alveoli with impaired diffusion, if any are present. Venous admixture is also referred to as *right-to-left shunt flow*.

268. The answer is D. *(West, 5/e, pp 22–26.)* End-pulmonary capillary blood normally reaches equilibrium with alveolar tensions of carbon dioxide, nitrogen, and oxygen. This is because the blood normally spends enough time in the pulmonary capillaries for these gases to reach equilibrium. If nitrous oxide (N_2O) is added to the inspired gas, it would also quickly reach equilibrium with pulmonary capillary blood. Oxygen takes longer than CO_2, N_2, or N_2O to reach equilibrium because a large amount of O_2 must diffuse into the blood to saturate the hemoglobin. In contrast, carbon monoxide, which is used at very low partial pressures to measure the diffusing capacity of the lung, does not have time to reach equilibrium in the time the blood spends in the pulmonary capillaries. This is because carbon monoxide so avidly binds to hemoglobin. The P_{CO} in the pulmonary capillary rises very slowly.

269. The answer is E. *(Berne, 3/e, pp 602–607.)* In the graph accompanying the question, curve B shows a depressed ventilatory response to elevation of P_{CO_2}. The response would be produced by central nervous system depressants such as barbiturates, benzodiazepines such as diazepam (Valium), and narcotics such as morphine, as well as by diminished alertness (sleep), which would reflect the overall level of activity in the reticular activating system of the brainstem. The sensitivity of the respiratory center to P_{CO_2} may be increased during exercise.

270. The answer is B. *(West, 12/e, pp 581–582, 584–585.)* Hypoxemia or a decreased arterial P_{O_2} stimulates the peripheral chemoreceptors in both the carotid and aortic bodies. Hypoxemia does not stimulate the central chemoreceptors. When Pa_{O_2} falls below about 60 mmHg, the chemoreceptor reflex mediated by the peripheral chemoreceptors in the carotid bodies causes ventilation to increase. The peripheral chemoreceptors also have an input into the vasomotor centers in the medulla. The net effect of hypoxemic stimulation of the peripheral chemoreceptors on the cardiovascular system is to cause a reflex increase in arterial blood pressure.

271. The answer is D. *(Berne, 3/e, pp 602–605. West, 12/e, pp 581–583.)* Stimulation of the peripheral chemoreceptors, particularly the carotid bodies, causes an increase in ventilation that results in a decrease in Pa_{CO_2} (termed *hyperventilation*). Stimulation of other receptors in the body both within the lungs and elsewhere can affect ventilation and can override the normal chemical control of ventilation, thus causing either hyper- or hypoventilation. Stimulation of peripheral pain receptors tends to cause hyperventilation, whereas stimulation of visceral pain receptors tends to cause hypoventilation. Stimulation of irritant receptors (also called *rapidly adapting receptors*) and J (juxtacapillary) receptors generally causes rapid, shallow breathing, which can result in hyperventilation. Intense stimulation of J receptors can cause apnea. However, stimulation of the pulmonary stretch receptors terminates inspiration and alone would not be expected to cause hyperventilation.

272. The answer is D. *(West, 12/e, pp 242–243.)* A Swan-Ganz catheter can be floated in the pulmonary artery to measure pulmonary artery systolic and diastolic pressures and, if advanced far enough, pulmonary capillary wedge pressure. Pulmonary capillary wedge pressure is substantially lower than the mean pressure in the pulmonary artery and is an indirect measure of pulmonary venous and left atrial pressures. The Swan-Ganz catheter would not sense the aortic pressure, which is an order of magnitude higher than the pulmonary artery pressure.

273–277. The answers are 273-A, 274-A, 275-D, 276-C, 277-B. *(Berne, 3/e, pp 590–594.)* The hemoglobin molecule consists of four globin chains, each of which contains one heme unit. Each heme contains one iron atom in the ferrous (Fe^{2+}) state and each can bind one O_2 molecule. The binding of an O_2 molecule to one heme facilitates the binding of O_2 to the others. This cooperative interaction results in the sigmoid shape of the normal oxyhemoglobin dissociation curve (curve N). As the Pa_{O_2} increases, the amount of O_2 bound to hemoglobin increases until the hemoglobin is saturated. The P_{O_2} at which the hemoglobin is 50 percent saturated with oxygen is called the P_{50}. In normal adult blood at pH 7.4 and 37°C, it is about 29 mmHg. The P_{50} is used as a measure of the affinity of hemoglobin for oxygen. Under different conditions, the oxyhemoglobin dissociation curve can be shifted to the left or right of normal (curve N); that is, the affinity of hemoglobin for O_2 can be increased or decreased.

The globin chains of adult hemoglobin consist of two α and two β chains. Fetal hemoglobin has two α and two γ chains. Because of this difference, fetal hemoglobin does not bind 2,3-DPG and the fetal oxyhemoglobin dissociation curve is therefore shifted to the left (curve A) compared with the adult curve. The higher affinity for O_2 of the fetal hemoglobin facilitates the extraction of O_2 by the fetus from the maternal blood.

Within the red blood cells, there is a high concentration of 2,3-diphosphoglycerate (2,3-DPG), which is formed from 1,3-DPG, a product of glycolysis. An increase in the amount of 2,3-DPG in the red cells causes the oxyhemoglobin dissociation curve to shift to the right. A decrease in 2,3-DPG shifts the curve to the left. During acclimatization to altitude, the concentration of 2,3-DPG increases, causing the curve to shift toward the right (curve C). When blood is stored, the amount of 2,3-DPG falls, which shifts the curve to the left and hinders unloading of O_2 (curve A).

In anemia (curve D), the hematocrit is reduced, thereby reducing the hemoglobin concentration and the oxygen capacity of the blood. The P_{50} is not different from that of normal blood but the oxygen content of the blood at any given P_{O_2} is less because of the decreased amount of hemoglobin.

Carbon monoxide (CO) binds to hemoglobin (HbCO) more than 200 times as avidly as oxygen. When CO binds to hemoglobin, it shifts the oxyhemoglobin dissociation curve to the left and makes it less sigmoid in shape (curve B). The presence of HbCO reduces the amount of hemoglobin available to bind to oxygen and the shift of the curve to the left hinders the unloading of the O_2 that does bind.

278–279. The answers are 278-B, 279-E. *(West, 5/e, pp 109–110, 148–150.)* If a person inhales to total lung capacity (TLC) and then performs a forced expiration, the initial expiratory flow will be effort-dependent; that is, the magnitude of the flow will depend on the expiratory force generated by the person. As the lung volume decreases, however, the flow becomes effort-independent; that is, no matter how much force is generated by the expiratory muscles, the flow rate remains constant. In an obstructive lung disease such as emphysema, peak expiratory flow is reduced and TLC and residual volume (RV) are increased (curve B). In curve C the effort-dependent flow is reduced but the effort-independent flow is normal. This curve is generated by a person making a reduced effort. In restrictive disease, TLC, RV, and peak flow are reduced (curve E). However, because compliance is reduced in restrictive disease, the flow at any given lung volume is slightly greater than normal. Curve D could be generated by a person with both obstructive and restrictive disease. The decreased compliance would reduce TLC and the increased airway resistance would decrease flow.

280–283. The answers are 280-G, 281-G, 282-D, 283-E. *(West, 5/e, pp 54–57, 131–135.)* A large intrapulmonary shunt causes a large $\dot{V}/\dot{Q}$ mismatch and a decreased Pa_{O_2}. The low Pa_{O_2} will stimulate the peripheral chemoreceptors, which, in turn, will increase ventilation, causing P_{CO_2} to decrease. The decrease in P_{CO_2} will result in a respiratory alkalosis, so pH will rise. The increase in pH will be blunted by a lactic acidosis that may occur as a result of the hypoxemia.

The low atmospheric pressures at high altitude will result in the inspiration of air that is low in oxygen. The decrease in the inspired P_{O_2} will result in hypoxemia, which will activate the peripheral chemoreceptors. This, in turn, will increase ventilation and cause P_{CO_2} to decrease. The decrease in P_{CO_2} will result in a respiratory alkalosis, so pH will rise. The increase in pH will be blunted by a lactic acidosis that may occur as a result of the hypoxemia.

Metabolic acidosis is defined as a reduction in pH due to a reduced bicarbonate concentration. When pH declines, both the central and peripheral chemoreceptors will be stimulated. Increased chemoreceptor activity will cause an increased ventilation, which will lead to a decrease in P_{CO_2} and an increase in P_{O_2}.

Respiratory arrest causes an increase in P_{CO_2} and a reduction in P_{O_2}. The high P_{CO_2} and the lactic acidosis that accompanies the hypoxia will lead to a decrease in pH.

Renal and Acid-Base Physiology

DIRECTIONS: Each question below contains five suggested responses. Select the **one best** response to each question.

284. The consumption of oxygen by the kidney

(A) decreases as blood flow increases
(B) is regulated by erythropoietin
(C) remains constant as blood flow increases
(D) directly reflects the level of sodium transport
(E) is greatest in the medulla

285. Which one of the following ions contributes to the anion gap?

(A) Potassium
(B) Chloride
(C) Bicarbonate
(D) Sodium
(E) Lactate

286. The graph below plots the reabsorption of glucose in the urine as a function of plasma glucose concentration. The renal threshold for glucose is located at point

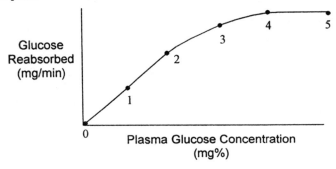

Glucose
Reabsorbed
(mg/min)

Plasma Glucose Concentration
(mg%)

(A) 1
(B) 2
(C) 3
(D) 4
(E) 5

---

287. In the presence of ADH, the filtrate will be isotonic to plasma in the

(A) descending limb of the loop of Henle
(B) ascending limb of the loop of Henle
(C) cortical collecting tubule
(D) medullary collecting tubule
(E) renal pelvis

288. Sodium reabsorption from the distal tubule will be increased if there is an increase in

(A) plasma potassium concentration
(B) plasma volume
(C) mean arterial pressure
(D) urine flow rate
(E) plasma osmolality

289. ADH will be released from the posterior pituitary when there is a decrease in

(A) plasma Na$^+$ concentration
(B) plasma volume
(C) plasma K$^+$ concentration
(D) plasma pH
(E) plasma Ca^{2+} concentration

290. If 600 mL of water is ingested rapidly, plasma volume will increase by approximately

(A) 400 mL
(B) 200 mL
(C) 100 mL
(D) 50 mL
(E) 25 mL

291. If the plasma concentration of a freely filterable substance that is neither secreted nor reabsorbed is 0.125 mg/mL, its urine concentration 25 mg/mL, and urine formation 1.0 mL/min, the glomerular filtration rate is

(A) 50 mL/min
(B) 125 mL/min
(C) 150 mL/min
(D) 200 mL/min
(E) 362 mL/min

292. An increase in the concentration of plasma potassium causes an increase in

(A) release of renin
(B) secretion of aldosterone
(C) secretion of ADH
(D) release of natriuretic hormone
(E) production of angiotensin II

293. Amino acids are almost completely reabsorbed from the glomerular filtrate via active transport in the

(A) proximal tubule
(B) loop of Henle
(C) distal tubule
(D) collecting duct
(E) renal pelvis

Questions 294–297

Use the Henderson equation or the Henderson-Hasselbalch equation to calculate the missing acid-base parameters.

294. Patient X was admitted to the hospital with a Pa_{CO_2} of 30 mmHg and an arterial $[H^+]$ of 50 nmol/L (pH 7.30). His plasma bicarbonate concentration is

(A) 7.2 mmol/L
(B) 14.4 mmol/L
(C) 30.0 mmol/L
(D) 40.0 mmol/L
(E) 62.5 mmol/L

295. Patient X from the previous question most likely has which of the following acid-base disorders?

(A) Metabolic acidosis
(B) Metabolic alkalosis
(C) Respiratory acidosis
(D) Respiratory alkalosis
(E) Mixed metabolic acidosis and respiratory acidosis

296. Patient Y has a Pa_{CO_2} of 30 mmHg and a plasma bicarbonate concentration of 22 mmol/L. What is her concentration of plasma hydrogen ion (pH)?

(A) 18 nmol/L; pH = 7.75
(B) 28 nmol/L; pH = 7.56
(C) 33 nmol/L; pH = 7.49
(D) 40 nmol/L; pH = 7.40
(E) 48 nmol/L; pH = 7.32

297. Patient Y from the previous question most likely has which of the following acid-base disorders?

(A) Metabolic acidosis
(B) Metabolic alkalosis
(C) Respiratory acidosis
(D) Respiratory alkalosis
(E) Mixed metabolic alkalosis and respiratory acidosis

298. The daily production of hydrogen ion from CO_2 is primarily buffered by

(A) extracellular bicarbonate
(B) red blood cell bicarbonate
(C) red blood cell hemoglobin
(D) plasma proteins
(E) plasma phosphate

299. Glomerular filtration rate would be increased by

(A) constriction of the afferent arteriole
(B) a decrease in afferent arteriolar pressure
(C) compression of the renal capsule
(D) a decrease in the concentration of plasma protein
(E) a decrease in renal blood flow

300. The following clinical laboratory data were obtained from a patient with diabetes mellitus: plasma $[Na^+] = 140$ meq/L; plasma $[K^+] = 7.0$ meq/L; plasma $[Cl^-] = 105$ meq/L; plasma $[HCO_3^-] = 6$ meq/L; arterial $[H^+] = 80$ neq/L; plasma [glucose] = 600 mg/dL. Calculate the anion gap.

(A) 12 meq/L
(B) 22 meq/L
(C) 29 meq/L
(D) 36 meq/L
(E) 42 meq/L

301. The secretion of H^+ in the proximal tubule is primarily associated with

(A) excretion of potassium ion
(B) excretion of hydrogen ion
(C) reabsorption of calcium ion
(D) reabsorption of bicarbonate ion
(E) reabsorption of phosphate ion

Questions 302–303

The following measurements are obtained from a patient: PAH clearance = 750 mL/min; plasma creatinine concentration = 0.8 mg/dL; urinary creatinine concentration = 66 mg/dL; urinary excretion = 2 mL/min; plasma glucose concentration = 120 mg/dL.

302. What is the patient's filtration fraction?

(A) 0.18
(B) 0.20
(C) 0.22
(D) 0.24
(E) 0.26

303. Approximately how much glucose is reabsorbed by this patient's kidneys?

(A) 0 mg/min
(B) 120 mg/min
(C) 165 mg/min
(D) 200 mg/min
(E) 320 mg/min

Questions 304–306

The following measurements are taken from a patient:

Urinary volume = 1.5 L/day
Urinary $[HCO_3^-]$ = 4 meq/L
Urinary titratable
    acids = 10 meq/L urine
Urinary $[NH_4^+]$ = 20 meq/L

304. What is the daily net acid excretion for this patient?

(A) 51 meq/day
(B) 39 meq/day
(C) 34 meq/day
(D) 30 meq/day
(E) 26 meq/day

305. How much new bicarbonate is being formed per day in this patient?

(A) 51 meq/day
(B) 39 meq/day
(C) 34 meq/day
(D) 30 meq/day
(E) 26 meq/day

306. Assuming production of a normal fixed acid load, what is this patient's acid-base status?

(A) Normal
(B) Respiratory acidosis
(C) Metabolic acidosis
(D) Respiratory alkalosis
(E) None of the above

307. The major source of the *total* daily acid load produced by the body is

(A) anaerobic metabolism
(B) aerobic metabolism
(C) phospholipid catabolism
(D) protein catabolism
(E) triglyceride catabolism

308. The following data are obtained: renal artery para-aminohippuric acid concentration (A_{PAH}) = 0.05 mg/mL; renal vein PAH concentration (V_{PAH}) = 0.005 mg/mL; urinary PAH concentration (U_{PAH}) = 20 mg/mL; urinary flow rate = 2 mL/min. Renal plasma flow is closest to

(A) 500 mL/min
(B) 600 mL/min
(C) 700 mL/min
(D) 800 mL/min
(E) 900 mL/min

309. If a substance appears in the renal artery but not in the renal vein,

(A) its clearance is equal to the glomerular filtration rate
(B) it must be reabsorbed by the kidney
(C) its urinary concentration must be higher than its plasma concentration
(D) its clearance is equal to the renal plasma flow
(E) it must be filtered by the kidney

310. A freely filterable substance that is neither reabsorbed nor secreted has a renal artery concentration of 12 mg/mL and a renal vein concentration of 9 mg/mL. Calculate the filtration fraction (GFR/RPF).

(A) 0.05
(B) 0.15
(C) 0.25
(D) 0.35
(E) 0.45

311. Destruction of the supraoptic nuclei of the brain will produce which of the following changes in urinary volume and concentration? (Assume that fluid intake equals fluid loss.)

(A) Increased urinary volume and a very dilute urine
(B) Increased urinary volume and a concentrated urine
(C) Decreased urinary volume and a very dilute urine
(D) Decreased urinary volume and a concentrated urine
(E) None of the above

312. Which one of the following returns closest to normal during chronic respiratory acidosis?

(A) Alveolar ventilation
(B) Arterial P_{CO_2}
(C) Arterial P_{O_2}
(D) Plasma concentration of bicarbonate
(E) Arterial concentration of hydrogen ion

313. The pH of the tubular fluid in the distal nephron can be lower than that in the proximal tubule because

(A) a greater sodium gradient can be established across the wall of the distal nephron than across the wall of the proximal tubule
(B) more buffer is present in the tubular fluid of the distal nephron than in the proximal tubule
(C) more hydrogen ion is secreted into the distal nephron than into the proximal tubule
(D) the brush border of the distal nephron contains more carbonic anhydrase than that of the proximal tubule
(E) the tight junctions of the distal nephron are less leaky to solute than those of the proximal tubule

314. Which of the following statements about renin is true?

(A) It is secreted by cells of the proximal tubule
(B) Its secretion leads to loss of sodium and water from plasma
(C) Its secretion is stimulated by increased mean renal arterial pressure
(D) It converts angiotensinogen to angiotensin I
(E) It converts angiotensin I to angiotensin II

315. A patient is found to have a urine creatinine concentration of 196 mg/mL; a plasma creatinine concentration of 1.4 mg/mL; and a urine flow of 1 mL/min. The creatinine clearance is

(A) 75 mL/min
(B) 98 mL/min
(C) 125 mL/min
(D) 140 mL/min
(E) 196 mL/min

316. Renal correction of hyperkalemia will result in

(A) alkalosis
(B) acidosis
(C) increased secretion of HCO_3^-
(D) increased secretion of H^+
(E) increased excretion of Na^+

317. In 1 h, 54 mL of urine is collected from a test subject. The concentration of para-aminohippuric acid (PAH) in the plasma is 0.02 mg/mL, and in the urine it is 14 mg/mL. What is the effective renal plasma flow (ERPF)?

(A) 31.1 mL/min
(B) 128 mL/min
(C) 278 mL/min
(D) 630 mL/min
(E) 771 mL/min

318. Most of the glucose that is filtered through the glomerulus undergoes reabsorption in the

(A) proximal tubule
(B) descending limb of the loop of Henle
(C) ascending limb of the loop of Henle
(D) distal tubule
(E) collecting duct

319. Which of the following structural features distinguishes the epithelial cells of the proximal tubule from those of the distal tubule?

(A) The distal tubule has a thicker basement membrane
(B) The proximal tubule has a thicker basement membrane
(C) The proximal tubule has a more extensive brush border
(D) The proximal tubule forms the juxtaglomerular apparatus
(E) The distal tubule has fewer tight intercellular junctions

320. Which of the following statements concerning the renal handling of proteins is correct?

(A) Proteins are more likely to be filtered if they are negatively charged than if they are uncharged
(B) Proteins can be filtered and secreted but not reabsorbed by the kidney
(C) Most of the protein excreted each day is derived from tubular secretion
(D) Protein excretion is directly related to plasma protein concentration
(E) Protein excretion is increased by sympathetic stimulation of the kidney

321. Glomerular filtration rate (GFR) and renal blood flow (RBF) will both be increased if

(A) the efferent and afferent arterioles are both dilated
(B) the efferent and afferent arterioles are both constricted
(C) only the afferent arteriole is constricted
(D) only the efferent arteriole is constricted
(E) the afferent arteriole is constricted and the efferent arteriole is dilated

322. A man drinks 2 L of water to replenish the fluids lost by sweating during a period of exercise. Compared with the situation prior to the period of sweating,

(A) his intracellular fluid will be hypertonic
(B) his extracellular fluid will be hypertonic
(C) his intracellular fluid volume will be greater
(D) his extracellular fluid volume will be greater
(E) his intracellular and extracellular fluid volumes will be unchanged

323. Ammonia is an effective and important urinary buffer for which of the following reasons?

(A) Its production in the kidney decreases during chronic acidosis
(B) The walls of the renal tubules are impermeable to NH_3
(C) The walls of the renal tubules are impermeable to NH_4^+
(D) Its acid-base reaction has a low pK_a
(E) None of the above

324. The amount of potassium excreted by the kidney will decrease if

(A) distal tubular flow increases
(B) circulating aldosterone levels increase
(C) dietary intake of potassium increases
(D) Na^+ reabsorption by the distal nephron decreases
(E) the excretion of organic ions increases

325. A respiratory acidosis that results in an increase in the concentration of hydrogen ion in arterial blood from 40 neq/L (pH 7.4) to 50 neq/L (pH 7.3) would

(A) stimulate the peripheral chemoreceptors
(B) decrease the amount of ammonium excreted in the urine
(C) inhibit the central chemoreceptors
(D) increase the pH of the urine
(E) decrease the concentration of HCO_3^- in arterial blood

326. Which of the following substances will be more concentrated at the end of the proximal tubule than at the beginning of the proximal tubule?

(A) Glucose
(B) Creatinine
(C) Sodium
(D) Bicarbonate
(E) Phosphate

327. When a person is dehydrated, hypotonic fluid will be found in the

(A) glomerular filtrate
(B) proximal tubule
(C) loop of Henle
(D) cortical collecting tubule
(E) distal collecting duct

328. The electrically neutral active transport of sodium from the lumen of the kidney occurs in the

(A) proximal tubule
(B) descending limb of the loop of Henle
(C) ascending limb of the loop of Henle
(D) cortical collecting duct
(E) medullary collecting duct

329. In metabolic acidosis caused by diabetic ketoacidosis, which of the following would be greater than normal?

(A) Concentration of plasma HCO_3^-
(B) Anion gap
(C) Arterial P_{CO_2}
(D) Plasma pH
(E) None of the above

330. Decreasing the resistance of the afferent arteriole in the glomerulus of the kidney will decrease

(A) the renal plasma flow
(B) the filtration fraction
(C) the oncotic pressure of the peritubular capillary blood
(D) the glomerular filtration rate
(E) none of the above

331. If GFR increases, proximal tubular reabsorption of salt and water will increase by a process called *glomerulotubular balance.* Contributions to this process include

(A) an increase in peritubular capillary hydrostatic pressure
(B) a decrease in peritubular sodium concentration
(C) an increase in peritubular oncotic pressure
(D) an increase in proximal tubular flow
(E) an increase in peritubular capillary flow

332. Renin release from the juxtaglomerular apparatus is inhibited by

(A) beta-adrenergic agonists
(B) prostaglandins
(C) aldosterone
(D) stimulation of the macula densa
(E) increased pressure within the afferent arterioles

333. Patients with renal insufficiency develop very high plasma concentrations of urea (uremia) because of

(A) an increased synthesis of urea by the liver
(B) an increased reabsorption of urea by the proximal tubules
(C) a decreased secretion of urea by the distal tubules
(D) a decreased glomerular filtration rate
(E) an increased renal blood flow

334. Which one of the following statements about aldosterone is correct?

(A) It produces its effect by activating cAMP
(B) It produces its effect by increasing distal tubular permeability to sodium
(C) It causes an increased reabsorption of hydrogen ion
(D) It has its main effect on the proximal tubule
(E) It is secreted in response to an increase in blood pressure

335. The effect of antidiuretic hormone (ADH) on the kidney is to

(A) increase the permeability of the distal nephron to water
(B) increase the glomerular filtration rate
(C) increase the excretion of Na^+
(D) increase the excretion of water
(E) increase the diameter of the renal artery

336. In the distal tubules, sodium reabsorption is increased directly by increased

(A) sympathetic nerve stimulation of the kidney
(B) atrial natriuretic hormone secretion
(C) antidiuretic hormone secretion
(D) aldosterone secretion
(E) angiotensin secretion

337. The ability of the kidney to excrete a concentrated urine will increase if

(A) the permeability of the proximal tubule to water decreases
(B) the rate of blood flow through the medulla decreases
(C) the rate of flow through the loop of Henle increases
(D) the activity of the Na-K pump in the loop of Henle decreases
(E) the permeability of the collecting duct to water decreases

338. The glomerular filtration rate will increase if

(A) circulating blood volume increases
(B) the afferent arteriolar resistance increases
(C) the efferent arteriolar resistance decreases
(D) the plasma protein concentration decreases
(E) urine flow through the urethra is blocked

DIRECTIONS: Each numbered question or incomplete statement below is NEGATIVELY phrased. Select the **one best** lettered response.

339. Metabolic alkalosis can be caused by all the following EXCEPT

(A) hyperaldosteronism
(B) hyperventilation
(C) hypokalemia
(D) volume depletion
(E) vomiting

340. The syndrome of inappropriate antidiuretic hormone secretion (SIADH) is caused by the excess release of ADH. SIADH will cause all the following to decrease EXCEPT

(A) concentration of plasma sodium
(B) intracellular volume
(C) urinary flow
(D) plasma oncotic pressure
(E) plasma osmolarity

341. All the following comparisons between the distal nephron and the proximal tubule are correct EXCEPT

(A) the distal nephron is less permeable to hydrogen ion than is the proximal tubule
(B) the distal nephron is more responsive to aldosterone than is the proximal tubule
(C) the distal nephron has a more negative intraluminal potential than does the proximal tubule
(D) the distal nephron secretes more potassium than does the proximal tubule
(E) the distal nephron secretes more hydrogen ion than does the proximal tubule

342. The hypothalamus will cause the release of ADH in response to all the following stimuli EXCEPT

(A) dehydration
(B) severe hemorrhage
(C) decreased blood osmolarity
(D) pain, anxiety, or surgical stress
(E) nicotine

343. H^+ secretion in the distal nephron is enhanced by all the following EXCEPT

(A) an increase in the level of plasma aldosterone
(B) an increase in the tubular luminal concentration of poorly reabsorbable anions
(C) hyperkalemia
(D) metabolic acidosis
(E) respiratory acidosis

344. In controlling the synthesis and secretion of aldosterone, which of the following factors is LEAST important?

(A) Renin
(B) Angiotensin II
(C) Circulating blood volume
(D) Concentration of plasma K^+
(E) Adrenocorticotropic hormone (ACTH)

345. Urinary volume is increased by all the following EXCEPT

(A) diabetes insipidus
(B) diabetes mellitus
(C) sympathetic stimulation
(D) increased renal arterial pressure
(E) infusion of mannitol

346. Significant buffers for hydrogen ions generated in the body from anaerobic metabolism include all the following EXCEPT

(A) extracellular bicarbonate
(B) plasma proteins
(C) plasma lactate
(D) inorganic phosphates
(E) intracellular proteins

347. Extracellular bicarbonate ions serve as an effective buffer for all the following EXCEPT

(A) sulfuric acid
(B) phosphoric acid
(C) lactic acid
(D) carbonic acid
(E) β-hydroxybutyric acid

348. All the following statements are true of the H^+ secreted into the lumen of the distal nephron EXCEPT that it

(A) can combine with NH_4^+
(B) can combine with HCO_3^-
(C) can combine with HPO_4^{2-}
(D) can remain as free H^+
(E) is secreted by an H^+-ATPase pump

349. During chronic metabolic acidosis, all the following will occur EXCEPT

(A) all the filtered HCO_3^- will be reabsorbed by the kidney
(B) the production of ammonia by the kidney will increase
(C) H^+ secretion in the distal nephron will be enhanced
(D) glutamine uptake by the kidney will be enhanced
(E) the urinary pH will be increased

350. In the presence of ADH, the cortical collecting tubule is LEAST permeable to

(A) water
(B) ammonia
(C) urea
(D) sodium
(E) carbon dioxide

351. The glomerular filtration barrier is composed of all the following EXCEPT

(A) fenestrated capillary endothelium
(B) macula densa
(C) basement membrane
(D) podocytes
(E) mesangial cells

352. All the following will cause an increase in reabsorption of bicarbonate in the kidney EXCEPT

(A) hyperaldosteronism
(B) hypercapnia
(C) hyperkalemia
(D) metabolic acidosis
(E) volume depletion

353. The amount of H^+ excreted as titratable acid bound to phosphate would be increased by all the following EXCEPT

(A) an increase in the amount of phosphate filtered at the glomerulus
(B) an increase in the pH of the urine
(C) an increase in the dietary intake of phosphate
(D) an increase in the level of plasma parathyroid hormone (PTH)
(E) a decrease in the renal tubular maximum (Tm) for phosphate reabsorption

354. Carbonic anhydrase plays an important role in all the following EXCEPT

(A) the renal handling of HCO_3^- within the cells of the proximal tubule
(B) the renal handling of HCO_3^- within the lumen of the proximal tubule
(C) the renal handling of HCO_3^- within the cells of the tubules of the distal nephron
(D) the renal handling of HCO_3^- within the lumen of the tubules of the distal nephron
(E) the gastric secretion of HCl by the parietal cells

355. All the following statements about the fluid flowing through the juxtamedullary nephrons in the presence of ADH are correct EXCEPT

(A) the fluid is isotonic to plasma when it enters the loop of Henle
(B) the fluid is hypertonic to plasma as it passes from the descending limb of the loop of Henle to the ascending limb
(C) the fluid is isotonic to plasma when it leaves the loop of Henle
(D) the fluid is isotonic to plasma when it enters the medullary collecting tubule
(E) the fluid is hypertonic when it is excreted by the nephron

DIRECTIONS: Each group of questions below consists of lettered choices followed by a set of numbered items. For each numbered item select the **one** lettered choice with which it is **most** closely associated. Each lettered choice may be used **once, more than once, or not at all**.

Questions 356–357

For each of the two conditions that follows, select the lettered point on the accompanying graph with which it is most likely to be associated.

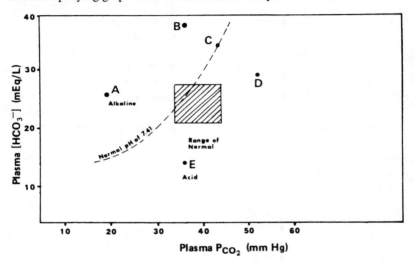

356. Uncompensated metabolic acidosis

357. Uncompensated respiratory alkalosis

Questions 358–359

The figure below shows the F/P ratio (the ratio of the concentration of a substance in the filtrate compared with the concentration of the substance in the plasma) for five freely filterable substances at various points along the proximal tubule. Choose the lettered substance for each question.

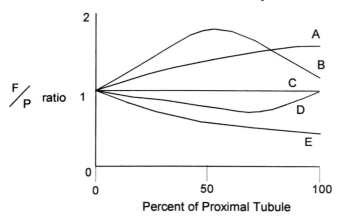

Percent of Proximal Tubule

358. For which substance is net reabsorption the lowest?

359. Which substance is most likely reabsorbed exclusively by solvent drag?

Questions 360–362

Which one of the substances below is described by each of the following statements?

(A) Aldosterone   (E) Atrial natriuretic hormone
(B) Parathyroid hormone   (F) Angiotensin
(C) Norepinephrine   (G) Prostaglandin
(D) Vasopressin   (H) Erythropoietin

360. It increases the renal clearance of phosphate

361. It increases glomerular filtration rate

362. It increases the water permeability of the collecting duct

Questions 363–365

For each of the following conditions, select the point on the accompanying graph with which it is most likely to be associated.

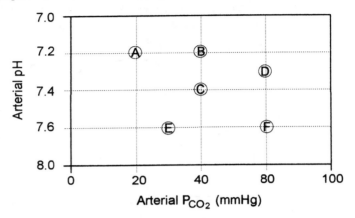

363. Metabolic acidosis

364. Respiratory acidosis

365. Ascent to high altitude

Questions 366–370

Match each of the descriptions below with the appropriate region of the kidney.

(A) Afferent arteriole
(B) Glomerulus
(C) Proximal tubule
(D) Descending limb of the loop of Henle
(E) Ascending limb of the loop of Henle
(F) Macula densa
(G) Vasa rectae
(H) Collecting duct

366. Isotonic reabsorption of sodium

367. Site at which permeability to water varies with plasma osmolarity

368. Site of the active transport system that makes it possible for the kidneys to excrete a concentrated urine

369. Site at which parathyroid hormone (PTH) regulates reabsorption of phosphate

370. A capillary network that is found only in the cortex of the kidney

Renal and Acid-Base Physiology

Answers

284. The answer is D. *(Ganong, 16/e, p 641. West, 12/e, p 436.)* In the kidney, oxygen is used primarily to support active transport of solutes, especially sodium, out of the tubules. In fact, oxygen consumption by the kidney is directly proportional to the amount of sodium reabsorbed and is greatest in the cortex, where most tubular reabsorption of sodium occurs. An increase in renal blood flow will raise the glomerular filtration rate and increase the quantity of solute to be transported, so that oxygen consumption increases as blood flow increases and the arteriovenous oxygen difference remains constant. This is in contrast to the situation in other organs where increases in blood flow are accompanied by a decrease in arteriovenous oxygen difference. Erythropoietin is released in response to renal hypoxia and acts to increase erythrocyte production.

285. The answer is E. *(Rose, 4/e, pp 545–551.)* The anion gap is calculated by subtracting the concentration of the major anions, chloride (Cl^-) and bicarbonate (HCO_3^-), from the sodium (Na^+) concentration. The difference represents the concentration of the minor anions (e.g., lactate, sulfate) in the plasma. The normal anion gap is about 8 to 12 meq/L. Increases in the anion gap occur with some types of metabolic acidosis such as diabetes and lactic acidosis but not with others such as loss of bicarbonate due to diarrhea or renal tubular acidosis.

286. The answer is C. *(Berne, 3/e, pp 729–731. Rose, 4/e, pp 84–86.)* As the plasma concentration of glucose increases, its filtered load (GFR $[Glucose]_{Plasma}$) increases linearly. At normal plasma glucose concentrations, the entire filtered load of glucose is reabsorbed and therefore the reabsorption of glucose also increases linearly as plasma glucose concentration increases (points 0 to 2). If the concentration of glucose continues to increase, the filtered load will exceed the reabsorptive capacity of the proximal tubule and therefore some of the glucose will not be reabsorbed (points 3 to 5). The plasma concentration at which glucose first appears in the urine (point 2) is called the *renal threshold* for glucose. The filtered load at this concentration is typically less than the transport maximum (T_M) for glucose. Thus the rate of reabsorption continues to rise as the plasma concentration rises until the filtered load reaches the T_M. This occurs at point 4.

287. The answer is C. *(Berne, 3/e, pp 762–770.)* In the absence of antidiuretic hormone (ADH, vasopressin), the cortical and medullary collecting tubules and ducts are impermeable to water. ADH increases the water permeability of these nephron segments and allows the filtrate to reach osmotic equilibrium with the interstitial fluid surrounding the nephron. The interstitial fluid in the cortex of the kidney is isotonic to plasma and therefore the filtrate can become isotonic to plasma in the cortical collecting tubule. The interstitial fluid is hypertonic to plasma in the medullary collecting tubule and so the filtrate becomes hypertonic to plasma in this region of the nephron and remains hypertonic as it passes through the renal pelvis. ADH has no effect on the water permeability of the loop of Henle. The filtrate is hypertonic to plasma in the descending limb and becomes hypotonic to plasma by the time it reaches the end of the ascending limb of the loop of Henle.

288. The answer is A. *(Berne, 3/e, pp 772–774, 785.)* Sodium (Na^+) reabsorption in the distal nephron is controlled primarily by aldosterone. Increases in plasma aldosterone concentration increase Na^+ reabsorption. Aldosterone secretion is increased when plasma concentrations of angiotensin II or potassium (K^+) are increased. Increases in plasma volume or mean arterial pressure will lead to a decrease in angiotensin II secretion. Increases in plasma osmolality will cause an increase in ADH. ADH will decrease water excretion but have only a minimal effect on sodium reabsorption. An increase in urinary flow rate may cause a slight decrease in sodium reabsorption.

289. The answer is B. *(Berne, 3/e, pp 758–762.)* Large amounts of antidiuretic hormone (ADH, vasopressin) are released from the posterior pituitary gland in response to a decrease in plasma volume or mean blood pressure. The increase in ADH helps to restore blood pressure by directly stimulating vascular smooth muscle and therefore increasing total peripheral resistance (TPR); it also helps to restore blood volume by decreasing the amount of water excreted by the kidneys. Osmoreceptors in the hypothalamus respond to a decrease in plasma osmolality by decreasing the amount of ADH secreted by the posterior pituitary gland.

290. The answer is D. *(Berne, 3/e, pp 754–758.)* When water is ingested from the intestine, it enters the plasma and rapidly achieves osmotic equilibrium with the interstitial and intracellular compartments. Since the plasma volume is approximately 8 percent (1/12) of the total body water volume, only 8 percent of the ingested water will remain in the plasma. Therefore, of the 600 mL of water ingested, approximately 50 mL remains in the plasma, 150 mL enters the interstitium, and 400 mL enters the intracellular space.

291. The answer is D. *(Ganong, 16/e, pp 641–642. Guyton, 8/e, pp 306–307.)* The glomerular filtration rate (GFR) is the volume of filtrate passing through all the nephrons each minute. It is influenced by the rate of blood flow through glomerular capillaries and by the permeability of the glomerular capillary wall and basement membrane. By using inulin, which is freely filtered and not reabsorbed or secreted, it is possible to determine the rate at which plasma passes through the glomerulus by comparing the rate of urinary excretion (urine volume times urinary concentration) with the plasma concentration, inasmuch as the filtered load equals the excreted load. Thus, for the example presented in the question,

$$\text{GFR} = \frac{25 \text{ mg/mL} \times 1 \text{ mL/min}}{0.125 \text{ mg/mL}} = 200 \text{ mL/min.}$$

292. The answer is B. *(Guyton, 8/e, pp 326–328.)* Aldosterone is the major hormone controlling the secretion of potassium by the distal tubule. It enhances the permeability of the luminal membrane to potassium, thus increasing the flow of potassium from the epithelial cells of the nephron, and increases the activity of the basolateral Na-K pump, thus increasing the movement of potassium from the interstitium to the epithelial cells. Potassium acts directly on the adrenal gland to increase the production and release of aldosterone.

293. The answer is A. *(Guyton, 8/e, pp 301–302.)* Amino acids are almost completely reabsorbed in the proximal renal tubules, along with glucose, proteins, acetoacetate ions, and vitamins. Very little of these substances is left in the tubular fluid entering the loop of Henle. Proteins, owing to their large size, are absorbed by pinocytosis through the proximal tubules' brush borders.

294–297. The answers are 294-B, 295-A, 296-C, 297-D. *(Berne, 3/e, pp 805–807. Rose, 4/e, pp 504–509.)* The Henderson and Henderson-Hasselbalch equations for the bicarbonate buffer system are used to evaluate acid-base status. The Henderson equation is

$$[\text{H}^+] \text{ (in nmol/L)} = 24 \times \frac{\text{Pa}_{\text{CO}_2} \text{ (in mmHg)}}{[\text{HCO}_3^-] \text{ (in mmol/L)}}$$

The conversion factors for the units and the K_a are "contained" in the number 24. The Henderson-Hasselbalch equation is the logarithmic form of this equation:

$$pH = 6.10 + \log \left(\frac{[HCO_3^-] \ (\text{in mmol/L})}{0.03 \ \dfrac{\text{mmol/L}}{\text{mmHg}} \times Pa_{CO_2} \ (\text{in mmHg})} \right)$$

The normal values are $[H^+] = 40$ nmol/L, pH $= 7.40$, $Pa_{CO_2} = 40$ mmHg, and $[HCO_3^-] = 24$ mmol/L. In practice it is easier to use the Henderson equation. For patient X the following would result:

$$50 \text{ nmol/L} = 24 \times \frac{30 \text{ mmHg}}{[HCO_3^-]}$$

$$[HCO_3^-] = 14.4 \text{ mmol/L}$$

Patient X has a higher-than-normal concentration of H^+ ion (a lower-than-normal pH). This indicates that an acidosis is present. He also has a lower-than-normal Pa_{CO_2}, which indicates he is hyperventilating. His bicarbonate level is also low. He most likely has a metabolic acidosis. Bicarbonate was consumed in the buffering of fixed acid. The Pa_{CO_2} is low because of stimulation of ventilation by the low arterial pH (respiratory compensation).

The following results can be obtained for patient Y:

$$[H^+] = 24 \times \frac{30 \text{ mmHg}}{22 \text{ mmol/L}}$$

$$[H^+] = 33 \text{ nmol/L (pH} = 7.49)$$

Patient Y has a lower-than-normal concentration of H^+ ion (higher-than-normal pH) and therefore has an alkalosis. Since the Pa_{CO_2} is lower than normal, the patient is hyperventilating and the alkalosis is therefore a respiratory alkalosis. The bicarbonate concentration is only slightly below normal and this reduction is due to the decrease in Pa_{CO_2} (acute respiratory alkalosis). Over time, if the hyperventilation continues, the kidneys would excrete bicarbonate and further reduce the plasma bicarbonate level to raise the arterial $[H^+]$ back toward normal (chronic respiratory alkalosis).

298. The answer is C. *(Berne, 3/e, pp 798–799. Rose, 4/e, pp 281–282, 287–289.)* Aerobic metabolism produces 13,000 to 24,000 mmol CO_2 per day. This yields close to that amount of H^+ ions produced per day via the reaction $CO_2 + H_2O \rightleftharpoons H_2CO_3 \rightleftharpoons H^+ + HCO_3^-$. At the tissues, CO_2 diffuses into the red cells, where the enzyme carbonic anhydrase accelerates the above reaction. The H^+ produced is buffered mainly by the large amount of hemoglobin in the red blood cells. Bicarbonate is not an effective buffer of volatile acid (from CO_2).

299. The answer is D. *(Ganong, 16/e, pp 641–644. Guyton, 8/e, pp 291–294.)* Glomerular filtration rate (GFR) will increase if there is an increase in the net glomerular capillary pressure or the flow of fluid through the glomerulus. The net glomerular capillary pressure (for Starling forces) is equal to the glomerular capillary pressure minus the sum of the plasma oncotic pressure and intrarenal pressure. Constriction of the afferent arteriole decreases glomerular capillary pressure while compression of the renal capsule increases the intrarenal pressure. Both of these will cause a decrease in GFR. In contrast, decreasing the concentration of plasma protein will decrease the plasma oncotic pressure and lead to an increase in GFR.

300. The answer is C. *(Rose, 4/e, pp 545–548.)* The anion gap is equal to the difference between the plasma concentration of sodium, the major cation in the plasma, and the sum of the concentrations of plasma chloride and bicarbonate, the major measured anions in the plasma.

$$\text{Anion gap} = [Na^+] - ([Cl^-] + [HCO_3^-])$$

$$= 140 \text{ meq/L} - (105 \text{ meq/L} + 6 \text{ meq/L})$$

$$= 29 \text{ meq/L}$$

The normal plasma concentrations of Na^+, Cl^-, and HCO_3^- are 140 meq/L, 105 meq/L, and 24 meq/L, respectively. The normal anion gap is from 9 to 14 meq/L. The anion gap is elevated when the concentration of unmeasured anions in the plasma increases—for example, in cases of metabolic acidosis such as diabetic ketoacidosis and lactic acidosis. It is not elevated in metabolic acidosis caused by diarrhea.

301. The answer is D. *(Berne, 3/e, pp 799–801.)* In the proximal tubule a large amount of H^+ ion is secreted into the tubule lumen via an Na^+/H^+ antiporter (exchanger). Most of this H^+ combines with bicarbonate ion in the tubular fluid to form CO_2 and water. The CO_2 diffuses into the proximal tubular cells, where the opposite reaction takes place to form H^+ and HCO_3^-. The HCO_3^- exits the cells on the basolateral side and enters the blood as reabsorbed bicarbonate. Carbonic anhydrase is located on the luminal surface of the cells as well as inside the cells to facilitate the above reactions.

302–303. The answers are 302-C, 303-D. *(Guyton, 8/e, pp 304–307.)* The filtration fraction is the fraction of plasma filtered from the plasma flowing through the kidney, or GFR/RPF. Renal plasma flow is equal to the clearance of PAH; GFR is equal to the clearance of creatinine. Clearance of creatinine can be calculated using the following formula:

$$C_{cr} = \frac{U_{cr} \times \dot{V}}{P_{cr}}$$

$$= \frac{66 \times 2}{0.8}$$

$$= 165 \text{ mL/min}$$

Thus the filtration fraction = 165/750 = 0.22. At glucose concentrations below 150 to 200 mg/dL, the kidneys will reabsorb all the glucose passing through the kidney. The filtered load of glucose = $P_{glu} \times$ GFR = 120 mg/dL $\times$ 165 mL/min = 198 mg/min. Since all of this will be reabsorbed, the kidneys reabsorb approximately 200 mg of glucose per minute.

304–306. The answers are 304-B, 305-B, 306-D. *(Guyton, 8/e, pp 335–339. Rose, 4/e, pp 303–307, 322–326.)* Net acid excretion is equal to the sum of the amount of titratable acids plus the amount of the ammonium ions minus the amount of bicarbonate ions contained in the volume of urine produced per day.

Net acid excretion = ([titratable acids] + $[NH_4^+]$ − $[HCO_3^-]$) $\times$ urine
volume per day
= (10 meq/L + 20 meq/L − 4 meq/L) $\times$ 1.5 L/day
= 39 meq/day

Acid is excreted in urine bound to titratable acids, principally phosphates, and bound to ammonia as NH_4^+. If bicarbonate is present in urine, its amount must be subtracted because a bicarbonate ion excreted in the urine means that a hydrogen ion was left behind in the body. Conversely, a net hydrogen ion excreted means that a bicarbonate ion was left behind in the body. Thus, net acid excretion is equal to new bicarbonate formation.

The normal fixed acid production is 70 to 100 meq/day. This is eliminated by the kidneys. This patient excreted only 39 meq H^+ per day and is therefore conserving hydrogen ions. He is also excreting HCO_3^- (retaining H^+) and must therefore be in a state of respiratory alkalosis. In respiratory and metabolic acidoses, the excretion of H^+ ion by the kidney is increased above normal and no bicarbonate ion is excreted in the urine.

307. The answer is B. *(Berne, 3/e, pp 798–799. Guyton, 8/e, pp 334–335.)* Acid is produced in the body as volatile acid and nonvolatile, or fixed, acid. Volatile acid is from the CO_2 produced by aerobic metabolism in the mitochondria. This amounts to 13,000 to 24,000 mmol CO_2 and consequently H^+

per day. $CO_2 + H_2O \rightleftharpoons H_2CO_3 \rightleftharpoons H^+ + HCO_3^-$. In the lungs this CO_2 is blown off, thus eliminating the bulk of acid produced in the body. The fixed acids produced from other reactions in the body such as anaerobic metabolism and phospholipid and protein catabolism amount to 70 to 100 mmol per day and are excreted by the kidneys.

308. The answer is E. *(Berne, 3/e, pp 729–733. Rose, 4/e, pp 57–58.)* The clearance of PAH is a good estimate of renal plasma flow (RPF) because, under normal circumstances, almost all (more than 90 percent) the PAH passing through the kidney is excreted. However, less than 90 percent of the PAH might be reabsorbed in a diseased kidney. An accurate measure of RPF can be obtained from the formula

$$RPF = \frac{U_{PAH} \times \dot{V}}{A_{PAH} - V_{PAH}}$$

309. The answer is E. *(Berne, 3/e, pp 727–731.)* If a substance disappears from the circulation during its passage through the kidney, it usually indicates that it has been totally secreted into the nephron. In this case its clearance will be equal to the RPF. If the substance is bound to plasma proteins, it can be secreted without being filtered. Even if it is entirely secreted by the kidney, its urinary concentration may be less than its plasma concentration if the urinary flow rate is very high.

310. The answer is C. *(Berne, 3/e, pp 727–729.)* Since the amount of fluid excreted by the kidney is only a small fraction of the renal plasma flow, the volume of fluid in the vein is essentially equal to that in the artery. Thus the difference in concentration must be due to the loss of solute. Since the material is neither reabsorbed nor secreted, its removal from the plasma must have been by glomerular filtration. Given that the filtered solute was 3 mg/mL and the renal artery concentration was 12 mg/mL, the fraction of solute filtered (and thus the fraction of solvent filtered) was 3/12 or 0.25.

311. The answer is A. *(Berne, 3/e, pp 923–928.)* Destruction of the supraoptic nuclei eliminates antidiuretic hormone (ADH) production. In the absence of ADH, the collecting ducts of the kidney would be impermeable to water and the final urine would be as dilute as the fluid leaving the ascending limb of the loop of Henle. In the absence of increased fluid intake, loss of water in excess of solute would result in increased osmolarity of body fluid. To maintain normal osmolarity, fluid intake must be increased. The increased fluid intake results in increased urinary volume because no water is conserved.

312. The answer is E. *(Berne, 3/e, pp 805–807. Rose, 4/e, p 613.)* Respiratory acidosis is caused by hypoventilation, i.e., a decrease in alveolar ventilation. When alveolar ventilation initially decreases (acute respiratory acidosis), arterial P_{CO_2} increases, arterial pH decreases (plasma [H^+] increases), and arterial P_{O_2} decreases. If the hypoventilation persists, the kidneys act to increase the concentration of plasma bicarbonate and excrete H^+ ions to bring the arterial concentration of hydrogen ion (pH) back toward or to normal. Alveolar ventilation, arterial P_{CO_2}, and arterial P_{O_2} remain abnormal.

313. The answer is E. *(Berne, 3/e, pp 799–804. Rose, 4/e, pp 308–310.)* The pH of the tubular fluid in the distal nephron can be lower than that in the proximal tubule because the tight junctions between the cells in the distal nephron are "tighter," or less leaky, than those in the proximal tubule. An H^+ ion gradient of only 10 to 1 (i.e., a minimum luminal pH of about 6.4) can be established in the proximal tubule, whereas an H^+ ion gradient of 1000 to 1 (i.e., a minimum luminal pH of 4.4) can be established in the distal nephron. Because of the tighter junctions, the distal nephron can also establish a greater sodium gradient. Even though the distal nephron can maintain a lower luminal pH, a lesser volume of H^+ ions is actually secreted than in the proximal tubule. The distal nephron, unlike the proximal tubule, does not have a true brush border and there is no carbonic anhydrase on the luminal surface of the cells as in the proximal tubule.

314. The answer is D. *(Berne, 3/e, pp 722–725, 772–774. Rose, 4/e, pp 31–33.)* Renin is secreted by the juxtaglomerular cells (near the afferent arterioles) in response to decreased renal arterial pressure. It acts on angiotensinogen to form angiotensin I. Angiotensin I is then converted to angiotensin II, a highly potent pressor agent that, despite a short half-life in humans, has numerous regulator functions, including the control of aldosterone secretion and sodium and water conservation.

315. The answer is D. *(Rose, 4/e, pp 38–39.)* The clearance of a substance by the kidney represents the volume of plasma from which the substance is completely removed, or cleared, per unit time. For creatinine,

$$\text{Creatinine clearance} = \frac{\text{Urine creatinine concentration} \times \text{urine flow}}{\text{Plasma creatinine concentration}}$$

$$= \frac{196 \text{ mg/mL} \times 1 \text{ mL/min}}{1.4 \text{ mg/mL}}$$

$$= 140 \text{ mL/min}.$$

Because creatinine tubular reabsorption and secretion are roughly equivalent, creatinine clearance may be regarded as a close approximation of glomerular filtration rate as measured more accurately with inulin.

316. The answer is B. *(Rose, 4/e, pp 769–773, 823–825.)* Hyperkalemia produces an increase in aldosterone secretion by the adrenal cortex. Aldosterone acts on the distal tubule to increase sodium reabsorption and decrease sodium excretion, as well as to enhance potassium secretion. When potassium excretion in the distal tubule is enhanced, hydrogen ion secretion, which also occurs in exchange for sodium resorption, is diminished. This reflects intracellular alkalosis, which occurs with hyperkalemia as cells lose hydrogen ion to take up potassium. As hydrogen ion secretion diminishes, hydrogen ion is retained and acidosis ensues.

317. The answer is D. *(Berne, 3/e, pp 731–733.)* Effective renal plasma flow (ERPF) can be measured by determining the amount of an inert substance (not metabolized or stored in the kidney) excreted in the urine per unit time divided by the difference in its concentration in renal arterial blood and renal venous blood. Para-aminohippuric acid (PAH) is filtered readily and is also secreted by the renal tubule so that less than 10 percent of the filtered load is present in blood leaving the kidney. Thus, since its renal venous concentration would be negligible and its peripheral venous concentration would be identical to renal arterial concentration, the clearance of PAH would be a close approximation of ERPF. In the example given in the question,

$$\text{ERPF} = \frac{\text{Concentration of PAH in urine} \times \text{urine flow rate}}{\text{Concentration of PAH in plasma}}$$

$$= \frac{14 \text{ mg/mL} \times 54 \text{ mL/60 min}}{0.02 \text{ mg/mL}}$$

$$= 630 \text{ mL/min.}$$

Actual renal plasma flow would then be

$$\frac{\text{ERPF}}{\text{PAH extraction}} = \frac{630 \text{ mL/min}}{0.9} = 700 \text{ mL/min}$$

and

$$\text{Renal blood flow} = \frac{\text{RPF}}{1 - \text{Hct}} = \frac{700 \text{ mL/min}}{0.55} = 1270 \text{ mL/min.}$$

318. The answer is A. (*Guyton, 8/e, pp 303–304. Rose, 4/e, pp 84–86.*) Glucose reabsorption employs an active transport mechanism located in the proximal tubule. The same mechanism also transports fructose, galactose, and xylose. Essentially all filtered glucose is reabsorbed, inasmuch as the transport maximum (Tm) for glucose (320 mg/min) is not exceeded in normal persons. In diabetes mellitus, hyperglycemia results in a tubular filtration load that exceeds the Tm, and glycosuria ensues.

319. The answer is C. (*Guyton, 8/e, pp 301–305.*) The major structural differences between epithelial cells of the proximal and distal tubules account for the fact that 65 percent of glomerular filtrate is reabsorbed in the proximal tubule and that the proximal tubule is more permeable to water. The proximal tubule has an extensive brush border composed of numerous microvilli, which markedly increase the surface area for reabsorption, and the tubule also has an extensive network of intracellular channels. The distal tubule has many more tight junctions between cells, which makes it less permeable to water. No significant difference in basement membrane thickness is observed between the proximal and distal tubules. The juxtaglomerular apparatus is formed by cells of the distal tubule lying adjacent to the afferent arteriole.

320. The answer is E. (*Berne, 3/e, p 745. West, 12/e, pp 429–430, 456.*) Approximately two-thirds of the 40 to 150 mg of protein excreted per day by the kidney is derived from plasma proteins. The remainder is derived from the tubular secretion of a mucoprotein, the Tamm-Horsfall protein that is present in tubular casts appearing in urinary sediment. Not all plasma proteins are filtered equally because glomerular permeability is related to molecular size and charge. The larger and negatively charged proteins are poorly filtered. Most of the filtered protein is reabsorbed in the proximal tubule unless the filtered load exceeds the tubular capacity. Such overload would occur following damage to the glomerular basement membrane and breakdown of normal barriers, or following an increase in the plasma concentration of a small protein, such as myoglobin. Protein excretion is also increased by sympathetic stimulation, such as that occurring during exercise. In this situation, renal vasoconstriction reduces the glomerular filtration rate, which, by increasing the transit time of glomerular filtrate, favors diffusion of proteins across the basement membrane.

321. The answer is A. (*Guyton, 8/e, pp 288–295. West, 12/e, pp 432–433.*) Renal blood flow is determined by the renal artery pressure and the resistance of the renal vascular bed. Decreasing the resistance of either the afferent or efferent arterioles could increase RBF. Alternatively, if the resistance of one of these vessels decreased more than the resistance of the other one increased,

RBF would also increase. Glomerular filtration rate will increase if glomerular capillary pressure increases. This can occur if the afferent arteriolar resistance decreases or if the efferent arteriolar resistance increases.

322. The answer is C. *(Berne, 3/e, pp 754–758. West, 12/e, pp 415–417.)* Sweat normally contains about 40 to 60 meq of sodium per liter of fluid. Thus, approximately 100 meq of sodium will be lost from the extracellular fluid during the exercise period, and when the lost water is replenished, the extracellular fluid will become hypotonic. The hypotonic extracellular fluid will equilibrate with the intracellular fluid and make it hypotonic as well. Because the extracellular fluid volume is dependent on the amount of sodium, the loss of sodium will result in a decreased extracellular fluid volume and an increased intracellular fluid volume after water is replaced.

323. The answer is C. *(Berne, 3/e, pp 802–804. Rose, 4/e, pp 314–318.)* Ammonia (NH_3) is produced from amino acids in the cells of the renal tubules (mainly the proximal tubules), and its rate of production increases during acidosis. This is important in acidosis because it increases the total amount of H^+ ion that can be excreted in a given volume of urine. The NH_3 freely diffuses into the tubular lumen, and because of the high pK_a (9.2) of the reaction, essentially all of it combines with H^+ to form NH_4^+. This maintains the driving force for more NH_3 to passively diffuse into the lumen. The NH_4^+ that is formed gets "trapped" in the tubules and excreted because the tubules are impermeable to this cation.

324. The answer is D. *(Berne, 3/e, pp 788–791. West, 12/e, pp 504–507.)* The amount of potassium excreted is controlled by the amount of potassium secreted by the distal tubule. Potassium secretion is a passive process that depends on the electrochemical gradient between the distal tubular cells and the tubular lumen and the permeability of the luminal cells to potassium. By inhibiting Na^+ reabsorption, the intraluminal potential becomes less negative and K^+ secretion is reduced. K^+-sparing diuretics such as amiloride act in this fashion. Aldosterone increases the intracellular potassium concentration by augmenting the activity of the Na-K pump and increasing the potassium permeability of the luminal membrane. Increasing dietary intake increases the plasma potassium concentration, which in turn stimulates aldosterone production. Although it is only a minor factor, increasing the rate of distal tubular flow increases secretion by maintaining a low potassium concentration within the filtrate and thus increasing the electrochemical gradient for potassium.

325. The answer is A. *(Berne, 3/e, pp 797–806.)* An increase in arterial concentration of hydrogen ion from a normal value of 40 neq/L (pH 7.4) to 50 neq/L (pH 7.3) would constitute an acidosis. Acidosis in arterial blood rapidly stimulates the peripheral chemoreceptors in the carotid and aortic bodies. If the acidosis is a respiratory acidosis (elevated Pa_{CO_2}), the central chemoreceptors would be stimulated, but since the defect (hypoventilation) would be in the respiratory system, no respiratory compensation could occur. When Pa_{CO_2} is increased, plasma concentration of HCO_3^- is increased. Renal compensation for the acidosis causes a further increase in plasma concentration of HCO_3^-. If the acidosis is a metabolic acidosis, it takes time for the concentration of hydrogen ion in the brain's extracellular fluid to rise because of the presence of the blood-brain barrier. Therefore, the central chemoreceptors are stimulated only in chronic metabolic acidosis. Acidosis increases the formation of NH_3 in the kidney and increases the excretion of H^+ ions as ammonium (NH_4^+) ions. As more H^+ is excreted, the pH of the urine is decreased.

326. The answer is B. *(West, 12/e, pp 436–438, 451–456.)* Sodium is isoosmotically reabsorbed from the proximal tubule; that is, when sodium is reabsorbed, water flows out of the proximal tubule to maintain a constant osmolarity. Thus, the concentration of sodium does not normally change as the filtrate flows through the proximal tubule. Since creatinine cannot be reabsorbed from the tubule, its concentration rises as water is reabsorbed. The concentrations of glucose, bicarbonate, and phosphate are all less at the end of the proximal tubule than at the beginning.

327. The answer is C. *(Berne, 3/e, pp 762–768.)* When a person is dehydrated, ADH secretion increases. In the presence of ADH, the cortical and medullary collecting tubules become permeable to water and the filtrate within these portions of the nephron reaches osmotic equilibrium with the interstitial fluid surrounding them. The ascending limb of the loop of Henle is not affected by ADH and so remains impermeable to water. As sodium and other electrolytes are reabsorbed from the ascending limb, its filtrate becomes hypotonic. The glomerular filtrate and proximal tubular fluid remain isotonic to plasma, which in the case of dehydration is higher than normal.

328. The answer is C. *(West, 12/e, pp 462–463.)* In the ascending limb of the loop of Henle, sodium is actively transported by a transporter that has one binding site for sodium, one binding site for potassium, and two binding sites for chloride. Thus the transport of sodium is electrically neutral. Electrically neutral sodium transport also occurs in the distal convoluted tubule and connecting segment by a carrier that binds both sodium and chloride. In all other segments of the nephron, however, sodium transport is electrogenic; that is, sodium is transported unaccompanied by a negatively charged chloride ion.

329. The answer is B. *(Berne, 3/e, pp 805–806. Rose, 4/e, pp 542–548.)* In diabetic ketoacidosis there is an increased production of acetoacetic and β-hydroxybutyric acids, which leads to an increase in plasma concentration of hydrogen ion. These fixed acids are buffered by all body buffers but mainly by bicarbonate. The concentration of plasma HCO_3^- is therefore below normal. The consumption of bicarbonate and the addition of the anions of the fixed acids to the plasma cause an elevation of the anion gap. The anion gap is equal to plasma $[Na^+]$ − (plasma $[HCO_3^-]$ + plasma $[Cl^-]$), and is normally about 12 to 15 meq/L. The acidosis would stimulate the carotid body chemoreceptors (and eventually the central chemoreceptors) to cause an increase in ventilation, which decreases arterial P_{CO_2}.

330. The answer is E. *(Guyton, 8/e, pp 290–295.)* The fraction of plasma filtered out of the glomerular capillaries (FF) is proportional to the glomerular capillary pressure and the renal plasma flow (RPF). Decreasing the resistance of the afferent arteriole increases both the RPF and the glomerular capillary pressure; thus, FF will be increased. Since a larger fraction of a larger RPF is filtered, glomerular filtration rate will be increased. Because a larger fraction of fluid is removed from the plasma, the oncotic pressure of the plasma flowing into the peritubular capillaries will be increased.

331. The answer is C. *(Berne, 3/e, pp 751, 776, Rose, 4/e, pp 79–81.)* When water is filtered across the glomerulus, the protein concentration (the oncotic pressure) within the capillaries increases, which in turn increases the efficiency by which water reabsorbed from the proximal tubule is returned to the circulatory system. If GFR increases, it results in a larger increase in oncotic pressure. This in turn increases the amount of water reabsorbed from the proximal tubule.

332. The answer is E. *(Berne, 3/e, pp 772–774. Rose, 4/e, pp 31–33.)* Juxtaglomerular (JG) cells are sensitive to changes in afferent arterial intraluminal pressure. Increased pressure within the afferent arteriole leads to a decrease in renin release, while decreased pressure tends to increase renin release. Angiotensin appears to inhibit renin release by initiating the flow of calcium into the JG cells. Renin release is increased in response to increased activity in the sympathetic neurons innervating the kidney. Prostaglandins, particularly PGI_2 and PGE_2, stimulate renin release. Stimulation of the macula densa leads to an increase in renin release, and although the mechanism is not fully understood, it appears that increased delivery of NaCl to the distal nephron is responsible for stimulating the macula densa. Aldosterone does not appear to have any direct effect on renin release.

333. The answer is D. *(Rose, 4/e, pp 56, 86. West, 12/e, pp 443, 457–458, 472–473.)* Most urea is synthesized in the liver. Its excretion is dependent on its concentration in plasma and the glomerular filtration rate (GFR) in the kidney. Approximately 50 to 60 percent of filtered plasma urea is passively reabsorbed in the proximal tubule at normal GFR. In renal insufficiency, in which GFR is decreased, less urea is filtered and therefore less urea is excreted. The decreased excretion of urea results in an increase in its plasma concentration.

334. The answer is B. *(Berne, 3/e, pp 773–774, 968–970. West, 12/e, pp 825–826, 830–831.)* Aldosterone binds to an intracellular receptor that causes an increased synthesis of a variety of proteins, including K^+ and Na^+ ion channels and Na-K ATPase, which together act to increase Na^+ reabsorption and K^+ secretion by the tubular cells of the distal nephron. H^+ secretion is also enhanced by aldosterone. Aldosterone secretion is stimulated by a decrease in blood volume (through the renin-angiotensin system) and by increased plasma K^+ concentrations. High blood pressure, if it has any effect on aldosterone, will cause a decrease in its secretion.

335. The answer is A. *(Berne, 3/e, pp 758–768, 925–928.)* The principal physiologic action of antidiuretic hormone (ADH) is to increase water retention by the kidney. The hormone acts on the distal nephron to increase its permeability so that water more readily enters the hypertonic interstitium of the renal pyramids. Thus, the concentration of solutes in the urine is increased. ADH increases Na^+ reabsorption so that the actual amount of Na^+ excreted is decreased. It also acts as a vasoconstrictor; hence, it is called *arginine vasopressin* (AVP). ADH has no effect on glomerular filtration rate, and because it increases water reabsorption, it would decrease urine formation.

336. The answer is D. *(Berne, 3/e, pp 772–780, 968–970. West, 12/e, pp 480–485.)* Sodium reabsorption in the distal tubule is primarily regulated by aldosterone. Increases in aldosterone increase Na^+ reabsorption. Antidiuretic hormone will increase Na^+ reabsorption by the collecting ducts. Neither sympathetic nerve stimulation nor angiotensin has a direct effect on the distal tubule, but both increase Na^+ reabsorption by the proximal tubule. Atrial natriuretic hormone (ANH, or ANP) increase Na^+ excretion.

337. The answer is B. *(Berne, 3/e, pp 762–768. West, 12/e, pp 470–476.)* The counter-current multiplier concentrates urine by establishing a medullary interstitium that is hypertonic to plasma. In the presence of ADH, the fluid in the collecting duct reaches osmotic equilibrium with the medullary interstitium and thus is excreted as a hypertonic fluid. Anything that reduces the medullary hypertonicity, such as increasing the flow of filtrate through the loop of Henle or deceasing the activity of the Na-K pump, will decrease the ability of the kidney to excrete a concentrated urine. If the permeability of the collecting duct to water is decreased, the urine's tonicity will be decreased.

338. The answer is D. *(West, 12/e, pp 429–434.)* The amount of fluid filtered by the glomerulus (the GFR) will increase if filtration pressure rises or plasma oncotic pressure decreases. A decrease in filtration will occur if the pressure within the kidney rises. Intrarenal pressure will increase if the urine is unable to flow through the urethra and backs up into the kidney. The kidney uses a variety of regulatory mechanisms to keep GFR constant when there is a change in renal perfusion pressure. For example, if an increase in circulating blood volume causes an increase in perfusion pressure, the afferent arteriole will constrict to keep renal blood flow and GFR at their normal levels. However, if the afferent arteriolar resistance increases without an increase in perfusion pressure, the pressure within the glomerulus will decrease and cause a decrease in GFR. A similar result will occur if the efferent arteriolar resistance falls.

339. The answer is B. *(Rose, 4/e, pp 516, 522–527.)* Metabolic alkalosis is caused by the loss of nonvolatile, or fixed, acid from the body. This can be by loss of H^+ from the gastrointestinal tract such as in vomiting of gastric acid. The loss of acid can also be from the kidneys. During volume depletion and hyperaldosteronism, plasma levels of aldosterone are elevated. Aldosterone, which increases renal sodium reabsorption, also increases renal H^+ secretion and excretion. During hypokalemia, K^+ moves out of cells in part in exchange for H^+ ions. This acidifies the renal tubular cells and increases renal H^+ secretion and excretion. Hyperventilation causes a respiratory alkalosis by decreasing arterial P_{CO_2} and results in the loss of volatile acid from the body.

340. The answer is B. *(Guyton, 8/e, pp 314–315.)* Antidiuretic hormone (ADH) increases the permeability of the distal nephron to water. In high concentrations it also has a vasopressor effect (from which its other name, *arginine vasopressin*, is obtained). The increase in water permeability increases the amount of water reabsorbed from the distal nephron, thus producing a large decrease in urinary flow and a large increase in urinary osmolarity. The excess reabsorption of water produces a decrease in concentration of plasma proteins (oncotic pressure), sodium, and osmolarity. The decrease in plasma osmolarity causes a flow of water from the extracellular to the intracellular compartment. Therefore, intracellular volume increases.

341. The answer is E. *(Rose, 4/e, pp 132–134, 136–142, 769–770.)* The distal nephron is less permeable to most solutes than is the proximal tubule because of the presence of large numbers of tight junctions connecting the epithelial cells to each other. Because of its low permeability, the reabsorption of sodium, under the influence of aldosterone, generates a much more negative diffusion potential than can be produced in the proximal tubule. The proximal tubule reabsorbs about 60 percent of the filtered load of potassium. Almost all the remainder is reabsorbed in the loop of Henle. As a result, the amount of potassium excretion necessary to maintain potassium balance depends on the amount secreted in the distal nephron. Although more of the hydrogen secreted by the distal nephron is excreted, the proximal tubule secretes more. Almost all the hydrogen secreted by the proximal tubule is reclaimed in the reabsorption of bicarbonate.

342. The answer is C. *(Berne, 3/e, pp 923–928.)* Release of antidiuretic hormone (ADH) is controlled primarily by osmotic stimulation of the supraoptic nuclei of the hypothalamus. Because the effect of ADH is conservation of water for the maintenance of normal osmolarity, it follows that an increase and not a decrease in blood osmolarity would evoke ADH release. The other major stimulus to ADH secretion is reduction of effective plasma volume. Dehydration and hemorrhage both represent situations in which extracellular fluid volume would be decreased and conservation of water required. Pain and other neural stimuli, as well as pharmacologic agents such as nicotine and acetylcholine, also can promote ADH release.

343. The answer is C. *(Rose, 4/e, pp 322–334.)* H^+ secretion in the distal nephron is enhanced by acidification of the cells of the tubules. This occurs during both metabolic and respiratory acidosis. It also occurs during hypokalemia as H^+ from outside the cells exchanges for K^+ from inside the cells. The opposite occurs in hyperkalemia. Thus, renal H^+ secretion is diminished in hyperkalemia. Aldosterone directly stimulates H^+ secretion by the distal nephron, and by strongly stimulating Na^+ reabsorption it also enhances the negative potential in the tubular lumen. Similarly, the presence of poorly reabsorbable anions in the lumen enhances the negative potential, and this negativity aids in the secretion of the H^+ cations into the lumen.

344. The answer is E. *(Berne, 3/e, pp 773–775, 969–970. West, 12/e, pp 481–483.)* The synthesis and secretion of aldosterone are dependent primarily upon the renin-angiotensin system. Increased potassium concentration directly stimulates aldosterone secretion. Increased circulating blood volume leads to a decrease in renin secretion and therefore a decrease in aldosterone secretion. The role of aldrenocorticotropic hormone (ACTH) in aldosterone synthesis and secretion is negligible.

345. The answer is C. *(Guyton, 8/e, pp 292–295, 308–309, 350–351.)* The rate of fluid volume excretion is influenced by the glomerular filtration rate (GFR) and the rate of tubular reabsorption. Increased renal arterial pressure increases urinary volume by increasing GFR, whereas sympathetic stimulation, by causing vasoconstriction, decreases both GFR and urinary volume. An increase in the filtered load of an osmotically active solute that is not reabsorbed, such as the nonmetabolized carbohydrate mannitol, or that is filtered in excess of the tubular capacity, such as glucose in diabetes mellitus, will decrease water resorption in parallel, and an osmotic diuresis will ensue. In diabetes insipidus, ADH secretion is markedly reduced or absent and water passes through the relatively impermeable collecting ducts without being reabsorbed.

346. The answer is C. *(Guyton, 8/e, pp 331–334. Rose, 4/e, pp 285–289.)* Lactic acid, a fixed acid, is the product of anaerobic metabolism. Hydrogen ions from fixed acids produced in the body, such as lactic acid and ketone acids, are buffered by all available body buffers. They are buffered principally by bicarbonate through the reaction $H^+ + HCO_3^- \rightleftharpoons H_2CO_3 \rightleftharpoons CO_2 + H_2O$. The CO_2 produced is eliminated by the lungs. H^+ is later excreted by the kidney and HCO_3^- is added back to the plasma. Other body buffers are plasma proteins and intracellular proteins, including hemoglobin and inorganic phosphates. Lactate would not be a significant buffer as the acid produced is lactic acid.

347. The answer is D. *(Guyton, 8/e, pp 321–334. Rose, 4/e, pp 285–289.)* The bicarbonate buffer system is of major importance in the buffering of fixed acids produced in the body, such as sulfuric acid, phosphoric acid, lactic acid, and ketone acids (e.g., β-hydroxybutyric acid). The reaction is $H^+ + HCO_3^- \rightleftharpoons H_2CO_3 \rightleftharpoons CO_2 + H_2O$. Bicarbonate is ineffective in buffering acid produced from CO_2, e.g., carbonic acid (H_2CO_3), because CO_2 is a product of the buffering reaction.

348. The answer is A. *(Guyton, 8/e, pp 336–340.)* H^+ is secreted into the lumen of the distal tubule by an electrogenic H^+ ion pump. This H^+ can combine with all available urinary buffers such as NH_3, phosphate, and bicarbonate or can remain as free H^+. The H^+ that combines with HCO_3^- forms CO_2, which diffuses back into the cells. The amount of free H^+ and H^+ bound to buffers is dependent on the amounts of the buffers present, the pK of the buffers, and the amount of H^+ secreted.

349. The answer is E. *(Guyton, 8/e, pp 337–340.)* During chronic metabolic acidosis, the kidney attempts to restore body pH back to normal by increasing H$^+$ ion excretion and reabsorbing all the bicarbonate filtered at the glomerulus. Secretion of H$^+$ into the tubular lumen by the cells of both the proximal and distal nephron is enhanced. This enhances bicarbonate reabsorption in the proximal tubule and H$^+$ excretion in the distal nephron. During acidosis, the rate of production of ammonia from glutamine by the kidney is increased, which allows more H$^+$ to be excreted in the urine as NH$_4^+$. With the increase in acid excretion, the pH of the urine is decreased.

350. The answer is C. *(Berne, 3/e, pp 758–762.)* Carbon dioxide and ammonia are lipid-soluble and thus able to cross all cell membranes. The ascending limb of the loop of Henle and, in the absence of ADH, the remainder of the distal nephron are impermeable to water. However, in the presence of ADH, water permeability of the distal nephron increases. The cortical and outer medullary collecting ducts are not permeable to urea, even in the presence of ADH.

351. The answer is B. *(Berne, 3/e, pp 722–724. West, 12/e, pp 422–424.)* The glomerular filtration barrier through which solutes and water must pass to move from plasma to Bowman's capsule is composed of three layers: the capillary endothelium, the basement membrane, and the epithelium lining the nephron. The capillary endothelial cells contain fenestrations, or pores, which have a mean diameter of 70 nm. The epithelial cells lining the nephron are called *podocytes* because of numerous pedicles, or foot processes, that make contact with the basement membrane of the glomerular capillaries. The mesangium is located between the capillaries and the nephron. It contains mesangial cells surrounded by a matrix composed of a basement membrane–like material. Some mesangial cells are primarily involved in phagocytosis, while others are contractile and may influence glomerular blood flow. The macula densa is part of the juxtaglomerular apparatus and is outside the glomerulus.

352. The answer is C. *(Berne, 3/e, pp 799–804. Rose, 4/e, pp 310–313.)* Filtered bicarbonate is reabsorbed in the kidney via an indirect mechanism that involves H$^+$ secretion into the lumen of the tubules. There, CO$_2$ is formed via the reaction H$^+$ + HCO$_3^-$ $\longrightarrow$ H$_2$CO$_3$ $\longrightarrow$ CO$_2$ + H$_2$O. CO$_2$ freely diffuses into the cells, where in the presence of carbonic anhydrase the reaction reverses and forms H$^+$, which can again be secreted, and HCO$_3^-$, which exits the cells on the peritubular side and is thereby reabsorbed. Intracellular acidification of the renal tubular cells that occurs during hypercapnia and metabolic acidosis causes an increase in secretion of H$^+$ ion and therefore an increase in reabsorption of bicarbonate. Hyperkalemia causes intracellular alkalinization via exchange of K$^+$ and H$^+$ and therefore would decrease H$^+$ secretion and decrease HCO$_3^-$ reabsorption. During volume depletion, there is an increase in the level of plasma aldosterone. Aldosterone stimulates H^+ secretion in the distal nephron, thereby increasing HCO_3^- reabsorption.

353. The answer is B. *(Berne, 3/e, pp 796–799. Rose, 4/e, pp 88–89, 314–315.)* Phosphate in plasma is freely filtered at the glomerulus. The amount filtered is dependent on the plasma level of phosphate, which is directly influenced by the amount of phosphate in the diet. No phosphate is secreted into the lumen of the renal tubules; however, phosphate in the form HPO_4^{2-} can be reabsorbed. The level of parathyroid hormone (PTH) helps control the amount of HPO_4^{2-} reabsorption. An increase in the plasma PTH level decreases the renal reabsorption of phosphate. Phosphate in the form $H_2PO_4^-$, which is more abundant at low pH levels, is not reabsorbed. Therefore, when the pH of the urine is low and more phosphate is in the form $H_2PO_4^-$, less phosphate can be reabsorbed, and more H^+ will be excreted in the urine bound to phosphate. Phosphate is reabsorbed via a carrier-mediated process that exhibits a tubular maximum (Tm). If the Tm is decreased, maximum reabsorption would be reached at a lower plasma phosphate concentration and more phosphate would be excreted.

354. The answer is D. *(Guyton, 8/e, pp 336–337. Rose, 4/e, pp 311–313.)* Carbonic anhydrase is the enzyme that catalyzes the following reaction: $CO_2 + H_2O \overset{CA}{\rightleftharpoons} H_2CO_3 \rightleftharpoons H^+ + HCO_3^-$. In the nephron it is located within tubular cells of both the proximal tubule and distal nephron (i.e., distal tubule, collecting tubule, and collecting duct), where it provides H^+ for secretion into the lumen and HCO_3^- for transport across the basolateral surfaces of the tubular cells. It is also located extracellularly on the brush border of the luminal surface of the cells of the proximal tubule S_1 and S_2 segments but is generally not located on the luminal surface of the cells of the distal nephron. In the proximal tubule, this luminal carbonic anhydrase catalyzes the formation of CO_2 and H_2O from H_2CO_3, which is in turn formed from filtered HCO_3^- and H^+ secreted into the lumen by the Na^+/H^+ exchanger of the cells of the proximal tubule. The CO_2 formed diffuses into the cells, where it can again form H^+ and HCO_3^- for secretion and reabsorption, respectively. The parietal cells of the gastric mucosa actively secrete HCl into the stomach cavity. The H^+ secreted and the HCO_3^- that is transported across the basolateral membrane of the cells are formed from the hydration of CO_2, catalyzed by the carbonic anhydrase within the parietal cells.

355. The answer is C. *(Berne, 3/e, pp 762–768. West, 12/e, pp 464–469.)* The filtrate remains isotonic as it passes through the proximal tubule and so it enters the loop of Henle as an isotonic fluid. As the filtrate flows through the descending limb of the loop of Henle, its tonicity increases as Na^+ enters and water leaves the filtrate. Na^+ is reabsorbed from the ascending limb, but because the ascending limb is impermeable to water, water does not follow and the filtrate leaving the loop of Henle becomes hypotonic to plasma. In the distal nephron, ADH causes the filtrate to become isotonic with the surrounding interstitium, which is isotonic to plasma in the cortex and hypertonic in the medulla. Thus, as the fluid passes through the cortical collecting duct, it becomes isotonic to plasma, and when it passes through the medullary collecting duct, it becomes hypertonic to plasma.

356–357. The answers are 356-E, 357-A. *(Berne, 3/e, pp 804–807. Guyton, 8/e, pp 340–343.)* Acid-base disturbances fall into four major groups that can be separated by examining their effects on the body's major buffer system — HCO_3^-/CO_2. Disturbances influencing one of these buffer substances will alter their ratio and alter pH.

Metabolic acidosis may result from (1) overproduction of organic acids such as acetoacetic acid in diabetes mellitus or lactic acid in hypoxia, (2) decreased renal excretion, or (3) drug ingestion. This increase in nonvolatile acid is neutralized by bicarbonate so that the net result is a decrease in bicarbonate without a change in P_{CO_2} (point E in the graph accompanying the question). Subsequent respiratory compensation would lower P_{CO_2}. In situations involving excess bicarbonate ingestion or acid loss (vomiting), the concentration of plasma HCO_3^- increases with no change in P_{CO_2}, and this produces metabolic alkalosis (point B). Subsequent respiratory compensation could cause a slight rise in P_{CO_2}.

Respiratory acidosis results from an increase in P_{CO_2}, which can be caused by primary pulmonary disease or any mechanism that compromises respiratory function and leads to CO_2 retention. In this condition, P_{CO_2} is increased with no acute change in concentration of HCO_3^- (point D). Hyperventilation, whether caused by voluntary action, exposure to altitude, or by disease of the central nervous system, promotes loss of CO_2 and lowers P_{CO_2}, with resultant respiratory alkalosis (point A).

The occurrence of each of these processes induces a compensatory response that attempts to restore the arterial pH to normal. In chronic respiratory acidosis, the kidney excretes hydrogen ion and acts to increase the plasma bicarbonate level to return the pH toward or to normal (point C). Arterial P_{CO_2} remains elevated. In many clinical situations, multiple acid-base disturbances may occur.

358–359. The answers are 358-A, 359-C. *(Guyton, 8/e, pp 303–305. Rose, 4/e, pp 67–68.)* Approximately 70 percent of the filtered water is normally reabsorbed from the proximal tubule. If less than 70 percent of a solute is reabsorbed in the proximal tubule, its F/P ratio (the ratio of the concentration of the substance in the filtrate to the concentration of the substance in the plasma) will rise as water is reabsorbed; if more than 70 percent of the solute is reabsorbed, its F/P ratio will fall. The F/P ratio of a substance can also increase if it is secreted into the proximal tubule. Substance A has the highest F/P ratio at the end of the proximal tubule and therefore has the lowest net reabsorption. The F/P ratio of substance B rose to a higher level than substance A by the middle of the proximal tubule, but fell to a lower F/P ratio at the end of the proximal tubule, indicating that most of its reabsorption occurred in the early portions of the proximal tubule. The F/P ratio of substance C did not change along the proximal tubule, indicating that it was reabsorbed at the same rate as water. This could occur in one of two ways. It could have been absorbed passively, like urea, by solvent drag. Or, like sodium (Na^+), it could have been reabsorbed actively. The F/P ratio of Na^+ does not change along the proximal tubule because water is drawn out of the proximal tubule by the osmotic pressure gradient established by the reabsorption of Na^+. Even though the F/P ratio of substance D at the end of the proximal tubule is the same as it is at the beginning, the decrease in its F/P ratio indicates that its reabsorption is at times greater than water and thus it could not be reabsorbed exclusively by solvent drag.

360–362. The answers are 360-B, 361-E, 362-D. *(Berne, 3/e, pp 758–762, 772–775, 795–797.)* Phosphate reabsorption is controlled by parathyroid hormone, which acts by inhibiting the sodium-dependent active transport of phosphate (HPO_4^{2-}). The control of phosphate reabsorption is indirect because parathyroid hormone secretion is stimulated by a decrease in plasma Ca^{2+} concentration. It is assumed that an abnormally high phosphate concentration will lead to a decrease in Ca^{2+} concentration and therefore an increase in parathyroid hormone secretion.

One of the ways in which atrial natriuretic hormone (ANH) increases sodium excretion is by increasing glomerular filtration rate (GFR). ANH increases GFR by dilating both the afferent and efferent arterioles.

Vasopressin (or antidiuretic hormone, ADH) increases water reabsorption from the distal nephron (the cortical and medullary collecting tubules and collecting ducts) by increasing the tubular permeability to water. It has no effect on water permeability of the proximal tubule, the loop of Henle, or the distal convoluted tubule.

363–365. The answers are 363-A, 364-D, 365-E. *(Berne, 3/e, pp 804–807.)* In metabolic acidosis there is an increase in the amount of fixed acids in the blood. This decreases arterial pH to a value lower than the normal value of 7.4 (point B). The low arterial pH stimulates carotid body chemoreceptors to increase ventilation, which results in a reduction of the arterial P_{CO_2} level below the normal value of 40 mmHg (point A). In respiratory acidosis, the primary disturbance is an increase in arterial P_{CO_2}, which results in a decrease in arterial pH (point D). The kidneys act to compensate by excreting hydrogen ions and increasing the plasma bicarbonate level. This brings the arterial pH back toward normal. At altitude, the reduction in arterial P_{O_2} that occurs as a result of the reduced barometric pressure stimulates the carotid body chemoreceptors to increase alveolar ventilation. The increase in alveolar ventilation decreases P_{CO_2} and causes an acute respiratory alkalosis (point E). With time, the kidneys act to excrete bicarbonate ion, which brings the arterial pH back toward normal.

366–370. The answers are 366-C, 367-H, 368-E, 369-C, 370-B. *(Berne, 3/e, pp 720–723, 741–743, 762–768, 795–797. West, 12/e, pp 425–426, 433–434, 456, 466–467, 481–482.)* In the proximal tubule, sodium diffuses passively across the luminal membrane of the epithelial cells and is then actively pumped out of the cell by an Na-K pump located on the basolateral surface. The presence of sodium in the basolateral spaces establishes an osmotic gradient, which causes water to flow out of the lumen. The flow of water down this osmotic gradient maintains the isotonicity of the filtrate and the reabsorbed fluid.

Antidiuretic hormone (ADH) regulates the osmolarity of the extracellular fluid by varying the permeability of the collecting duct to water. The increase in permeability to water caused by ADH allows water to flow out of the collecting duct down an osmotic gradient between the lumen and the medullary interstitium.

The high osmolarity of the medullary interstitium is created by the countercurrent multiplication system of the loop of Henle. The active transport process responsible for the countercurrent multiplier (a carrier that transports one ion of Na$^+$, one ion of K$^+$, and two ions of Cl$^-$) is located on the thick portion of the ascending limb of the loop of Henle.

PTH regulates the extracellular concentration of calcium and phosphate ions. In the kidney, it binds to a receptor on the basolateral surface of the epithelial cells of the proximal tubule and causes a decrease in reabsorption of phosphate.

The proximal tubule is the site of reabsorption of glucose (via secondary active transport). Glucose enters the tubular cells on a carrier that also binds sodium. The sodium that enters is then pumped out of the cell on the basolateral side by Na,K-ATPase.

The path of blood flow at the level of the nephron is first through the afferent arteriole and then through the glomerulus, which is composed of a capillary tuft found only in the cortex of the kidney. Blood from the glomerulus flows through the efferent arteriole into the peritubular capillaries. The vasa rectae are a capillary network found in the medulla of the kidney in association with the loop of Henle. They help to maintain the high medullary interstitial osmolarity established by the countercurrent multiplication system.

The smooth muscle of the afferent arteriole is the site of myogenic autoregulation of renal blood flow. An increase in blood pressure causes a constriction of the afferent arteriole. The aim of this mechanism is to maintain renal blood flow and glomerular filtration at constant rates.

The afferent arteriole in apposition to the beginning of the distal tubule forms the juxtaglomerular apparatus (JGA). This consists of the macula densa, which is composed of specialized cells of the distal tubule, and the juxtaglomerular (or granular) cells, which are specialized cells of the walls of the afferent arteriole. In the juxtaglomerular cells are granules containing the enzyme renin, which, when released into the blood, converts angiotensinogen (renin substrate) to angiotensin I.

Aldosterone is a hormone released by the zona glomerulosa of the adrenal cortex. An increase in aldosterone causes an increase in the reabsorption of sodium by the cells of the collecting duct by increasing sodium entry into the cells. The sodium is then pumped out via the Na,K-ATPase.

Endocrine Physiology

DIRECTIONS: Each question below contains five suggested responses. Select the **one best** response to each question.

371. The supraoptic nucleus of the hypothalamus is believed to control secretion of which of the following hormones?

(A) Antidiuretic hormone (arginine vasopressin)
(B) Oxytocin
(C) Growth hormone
(D) Adrenocorticotropic hormone
(E) Follicle-stimulating hormone

372. Parathyroid hormone (PTH) is accurately described by which of the following statements?

(A) It is secreted in response to an increase in plasma Ca^{2+} concentration
(B) It acts directly on bone cells to increase Ca^{2+} deposition
(C) It acts directly on intestinal cells to increase Ca^{2+} absorption
(D) It causes a decrease in cAMP concentration within renal proximal tubular cells
(E) It is essential for life

373. When a person is in the fasting state,

(A) liver glycogen levels are increased
(B) the excretion of urea in the urine decreases
(C) basal metabolic rate (BMR) decreases
(D) glucose is the only fuel used by the central nervous system
(E) gluconeogenesis is inhibited

374. True statements regarding atrial natriuretic hormone (ANH) include that it

(A) is synthesized from cholesterol
(B) is secreted in response to hypovolemia
(C) increases total peripheral resistance
(D) decreases glomerular filtration rate
(E) inhibits aldosterone secretion

375. Which one of the following statements about spermatogenesis is correct?

(A) Production and release of spermatozoa is cyclical
(B) Sertoli cells are required for mitotic and meiotic activity of germ cells
(C) Spermatogenesis requires continuous release of gonadotropin-releasing hormone (GRH)
(D) Leydig cell secretion of testosterone requires follicle-stimulating hormone (FSH)
(E) Luteinizing hormone (LH) acts directly on Sertoli cells to promote cell division

376. The secretion of growth hormone is increased by

(A) hyperglycemia
(B) exercise
(C) somatostatin
(D) growth hormone
(E) free fatty acids

377. In a woman with a regular menstrual cycle of 28 to 30 days, ovulation would be expected to occur between cycle days

(A) 6 and 8
(B) 10 and 12
(C) 14 and 16
(D) 18 and 20
(E) 22 and 24

378. Which one of the following hormones is secreted by the posterior pituitary gland?

(A) Adrenocorticotropic hormone (ACTH)
(B) Oxytocin
(C) Thyroid-stimulating hormone (TSH)
(D) Growth hormone (GH)
(E) Prolactin

379. Which one of the following statements about prolactin is correct?

(A) Prolactin initiates ovulation
(B) Prolactin causes milk ejection during suckling
(C) Prolactin inhibits the growth of breast tissue
(D) Prolactin secretion is tonically inhibited by the hypothalamus
(E) Prolactin secretion is increased by dopamine

380. The principal steroid secreted by the fetal adrenal cortex is

(A) cortisol
(B) corticosterone
(C) dehydroepiandrosterone
(D) progesterone
(E) pregnenolone

381. The effect of insulin on glucose transport is to

(A) permit transport against a concentration gradient
(B) enhance transport across the cell membrane
(C) enhance transport across the tubular epithelium of the kidney
(D) enhance transport into the brain
(E) enhance transport through the intestinal mucosa

382. Compared with the resting state, during prolonged exercise the caloric needs of skeletal muscle are met by

(A) release of free fatty acids from adipose tissue
(B) an increase in hepatic glycogenolysis
(C) an increase in gluconeogenesis in muscle
(D) increased intestinal uptake of glucose and amino acids
(E) none of the above

383. Administration of pharmacologic doses of aldosterone to a dog will have which of the following effects upon blood pressure (BP), body weight (BW), and plasma potassium (PP) levels?

	BP	BW	PP
(A)	Increased	Decreased	Increased
(B)	Increased	Increased	Decreased
(C)	Increased	Decreased	Decreased
(D)	Decreased	Increased	Decreased
(E)	Decreased	Decreased	Increased

384. The graph below demonstrates diurnal variation in the plasma level of

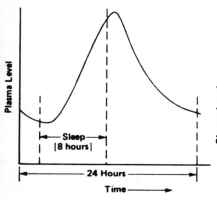

(A) thyroxine
(B) insulin
(C) parathyroid hormone
(D) cortisol
(E) estrogen

385. In the graph below, which shows plasma hormone levels as a function of time, ovulation takes place at which of the lettered points on the time axis?

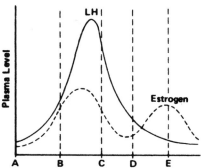

(A) A
(B) B
(C) C
(D) D
(E) E

386. Iodides are stored in the thyroid follicles mainly in the form of

(A) thyroxine
(B) thyroglobulin
(C) monoiodotyrosine
(D) diiodotyrosine
(E) 3,5,3'-triiodothyronine

387. The normal pattern of progesterone secretion during the menstrual cycle is exhibited by which of the curves shown below?

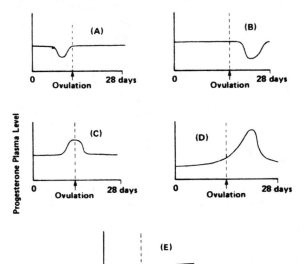

(A) A
(B) B
(C) C
(D) D
(E) E

---

388. Almost all the active thyroid hormone entering the circulation is in the form of

(A) triiodothyronine
(B) thyroxine
(C) thyroglobulin
(D) thyrotropin
(E) long-acting thyroid stimulator (LATS)

389. Physiologically active thyroxine exists in which of the following forms?

(A) Bound to albumin
(B) Bound to prealbumin
(C) Bound to globulin
(D) As a glucuronide
(E) Unbound

390. Which one of the following hormones is primarily responsible for the development of ovarian follicles prior to ovulation?

(A) Chorionic gonadotropin (hCG)
(B) Estradiol
(C) Follicle-stimulating hormone (FSH)
(D) Luteinizing hormone (LH)
(E) Progesterone

391. In the graph below of changes in endometrial thickness during a normal 28-day menstrual cycle, the event designated "A" corresponds most closely to

(A) the menstrual phase
(B) the maturation of the corpus luteum
(C) the early proliferative phase
(D) the secretory phase
(E) ovulation

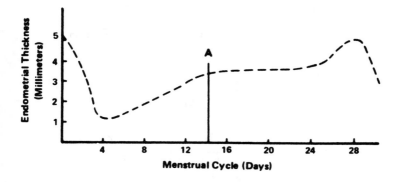

392. In a normal pregnancy, human chorionic gonadotropin (hCG) prevents the involution of the corpus luteum that normally occurs at the end of the menstrual cycle. Which of the curves shown below approximates the level of this hormone during pregnancy?

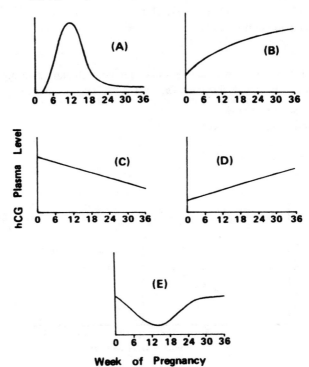

(A) A
(B) B
(C) C
(D) D
(E) E

393. Interaction of insulin with its membrane receptor

(A) affects transmembrane ion transport
(B) inhibits tyrosine phosphorylation in the receptor molecule
(C) reduces cellular glucose uptake
(D) results in enhanced binding of additional insulin molecules
(E) stimulates the synthesis of additional receptor molecules

394. Activation of hormone-sensitive lipase in adipocytes

(A) causes increased hydrolysis of cholesterol esters
(B) is mediated by a cyclic AMP–dependent protein kinase
(C) is prevented by cortisol
(D) is stimulated by insulin
(E) results in accumulation of monoglycerides and diglycerides in adipocytes

395. Which of the following is a correct statement about the production of human sperm?

(A) Spermatogonia undergo meiosis
(B) Spermatogenesis occurs in the epididymus
(C) Normally, 10 to 20 million sperm are produced daily
(D) FSH is required
(E) Complete maturation of spermatozoa occurs in 28 to 30 days

396. Functions of the Sertoli cells in the seminiferous tubules include

(A) secretion of FSH into the tubular lumen
(B) secretion of testosterone into the tubular lumen
(C) maintenance of the blood-testis barrier
(D) synthesis of estrogen after puberty
(E) none of the above

397. Which of the following statements about iron absorption and metabolism is correct?

(A) About 100 mg of iron is absorbed per day
(B) Iron is absorbed at a rapid rate from the intestine
(C) Iron in the blood is bound to transferrin
(D) Iron ingested in the ferrous state must, in general, be oxidized to the ferric state for absorption
(E) Iron absorption is a passive process regulated by circulating plasma iron levels

398. The islets of Langerhans are characterized by

(A) being more plentiful in the head of the pancreas than in the tail
(B) constituting 20 to 30 percent of the weight of the pancreas
(C) containing at least six distinct cell types
(D) having a meager blood supply
(E) producing glucagon and insulin

399. Plasma levels of calcium can be increased most rapidly by the direct action of parathyroid hormone on the

(A) kidney
(B) intestine
(C) thyroid gland
(D) bones
(E) skeletal musculature

400. Hyperparathyroidism is reflected in decreased plasma levels of

(A) phosphate
(B) sodium
(C) calcium
(D) potassium
(E) calcitonin

401. Correct statements about human growth hormone include which of the following?

(A) It is synthesized in the hypothalamus
(B) It stimulates production of somatomedins by the liver
(C) Its release is stimulated by somatostatin
(D) It causes a decrease in lipolysis
(E) None of the above

402. The basic effects of growth hormone on body metabolism include

(A) decreasing the rate of protein synthesis
(B) increasing the rate of use of carbohydrate
(C) decreasing the mobilization of fats
(D) increasing the use of fats for energy
(E) none of the above

403. Which of the following is true about the actions of glucagon?

(A) It stimulates glycogenolysis in muscle
(B) It inhibits insulin secretion
(C) It stimulates gluconeogenesis in the liver
(D) It inhibits adenyl cyclase
(E) It inhibits phospholipase C

404. One of the most common signs of hypoparathyroidism is

(A) phosphaturia
(B) hypercalcemia
(C) demineralization of bones
(D) hyperexcitability of muscles
(E) formation of kidney stones

405. Hormonal changes during normal pregnancy are correctly described by which one of the following statements?

(A) Estriol excretion is greatest just before parturition
(B) Human chorionic gonadotropin secretion is greatest in the third trimester
(C) Human chorionic somatomammotropin secretion is greatest in the first trimester
(D) Oxytocin secretion is greatest in the second trimester
(E) Pregnanediol excretion is greatest in the first trimester

406. Proinsulin is correctly described in which one of the following statements?

(A) It is a biosynthetic precursor of insulin
(B) It is cleaved by an enzyme on the cell surface
(C) It is a double-chain polypeptide
(D) It is the major form of insulin secreted by the pancreatic β cells
(E) It is more active than insulin on its target tissues

407. The actions of insulin include

(A) converting glycogen to glucose
(B) stimulating gluconeogenesis
(C) increasing plasma amino acid concentration
(D) enhancing potassium entry into cells
(E) reducing urine formation

408. The secretion of ACTH is correctly described in which of the following statements?

(A) It shows circadian rhythm in humans
(B) It is decreased during periods of stress
(C) It is inhibited by aldosterone
(D) It is stimulated by glucocorticoids
(E) It is stimulated by epinephrine

DIRECTIONS: Each numbered question or incomplete statement below is NEGATIVELY phrased. Select the **one best** lettered response.

409. Injection of thyroid hormone into a normal laboratory animal will produce all the following effects EXCEPT

(A) an increase in the rate of oxygen consumption
(B) an increase in the rate of muscle protein synthesis
(C) an increase in the need for vitamins
(D) a decrease in the plasma concentration of cholesterol
(E) a decrease in the rate of lipolysis

410. All the following are effects of primary hyperaldosteronism (Conn's syndrome) EXCEPT

(A) hypertension
(B) hyperkalemia
(C) expanded extracellular fluid volume
(D) decreased concentrating ability of the kidney
(E) decreased hematocrit

411. The adrenal cortex secretes all the following hormones EXCEPT

(A) epinephrine
(B) cortisol
(C) dehydroepiandrosterone (DHEA)
(D) aldosterone
(E) corticosterone

412. Removal of the adrenal glands generally has all the following consequences EXCEPT

(A) a tendency to hyperglycemia with decreased insulin sensitivity
(B) poor mobilization and utilization of fatty tissues
(C) poor water excretion by the kidneys and sodium loss in the urine
(D) poor resistance to infection or shock
(E) psychic changes such as depression or decreased alertness

413. All the following are characteristic of hyperparathyroidism EXCEPT

(A) demineralization of bone
(B) formation of kidney stones
(C) hypercalcemia
(D) hypercalciuria
(E) hyperphosphatemia

414. Insulin increases glucose uptake in all the following structures EXCEPT

(A) adipose tissue
(B) cardiac muscle
(C) skeletal muscle
(D) intestinal mucosa
(E) the uterus

415. Hyperglycemia is induced by all the following hormones EXCEPT

(A) epinephrine
(B) thyroxine
(C) ACTH
(D) glucagon
(E) aldosterone

416. The actions of angiotensin II include all the following EXCEPT

(A) direct constriction of peripheral arterioles
(B) promotion of salt excretion by renal tubules
(C) stimulation of aldosterone secretion
(D) inhibition of renin secretion
(E) stimulation of the subfornical organ of the diencephalon to promote drinking

417. All the following are characteristic of hypothyroidism EXCEPT

(A) bradycardia
(B) decreased metabolic rate
(C) heat intolerance
(D) sleepiness
(E) weight gain

418. Goiter (enlargement of the thyroid) can occur as a consequence of all the following EXCEPT

(A) iodine deficiency
(B) pituitary adenoma
(C) Graves' disease
(D) excessive intake of exogenous thyroxine
(E) excessive intake of cabbage and turnips

419. Secretion of growth hormone is stimulated by all the following EXCEPT

(A) L-arginine
(B) deep sleep
(C) free fatty acids
(D) growth hormone–releasing hormone (GRH)
(E) hypoglycemia

420. The basal metabolic rate (BMR) increases with all the following EXCEPT

(A) advancing age
(B) anxiety
(C) body surface area
(D) increased environmental temperature
(E) reduced environmental temperature

421. All the following statements about the uptake of triglycerides into adipose tissue from plasma lipoproteins are true EXCEPT

(A) it is regulated by the activity of lipoprotein lipase
(B) it is decreased by catecholamines
(C) it is increased by glucose
(D) it is increased by insulin
(E) it requires receptor-mediated endocytosis

422. True statements about implantation of the zygote in the uterus include all the following EXCEPT

(A) it follows dissolution of the zona pellucida
(B) it involves infiltration of the endometrium by the syncytiotrophoblast
(C) it occurs 6 to 7 days after fertilization
(D) it occurs when the embryo consists of approximately 32 cells
(E) it requires secretion of progesterone by the corpus luteum

423. An exceptionally muscular female athlete at an international athletic competition is noted to have increased facial hair and frontal balding. She should be evaluated for all the following EXCEPT

(A) an adrenal tumor
(B) an ovarian tumor
(C) deficiency of 11β-hydroxylase
(D) familial hyperlipoproteinemia
(E) use of synthetic androgens

424. Thyroxine and triiodothyronine are transported in plasma in all the following forms EXCEPT

(A) bound to thyroxine-binding globulin (TBG)
(B) bound to albumin
(C) bound to thyroxine-binding prealbumin (TBPA)
(D) bound to thyroglobulin
(E) as free hormones

425. Thyroid hormones exhibit all the following characteristics EXCEPT

(A) they display a long duration of activity
(B) injected thyroxine raises the metabolic rate within 24 h
(C) they are stored in extracellular sites
(D) they are transported by carrier proteins
(E) they affect the metabolism of most tissues of the body

426. Melatonin is correctly described by all the following statements EXCEPT

(A) it is synthesized from tryptophan
(B) it regulates skin pigmentation in humans
(C) its secretion is increased by darkness
(D) its secretion is stimulated by norepinephrine from the sympathetic nervous system
(E) reduction of its normal secretion by pineal tumors may cause premature puberty

427. Insulin deficiency leads to increaed use of fat as a result of all the following EXCEPT

(A) decreased cellular uptake of glucose
(B) decreased intracellular α-glycerophosphate in liver and fat cells
(C) exclusion of use of glucose except by brain tissue
(D) increased fatty acid release from adipose tissue
(E) indirect depression of use of glucose by excess fatty acids in the blood

428. Secretion of insulin is affected by all the following EXCEPT

(A) blood glucose
(B) Ca^{2+} and K^+ concentrations
(C) 2-deoxyglucose
(D) mannitol
(E) somatostatin

429. Correct statements about progesterone include all the following EXCEPT

(A) it is secreted by the corpus luteum
(B) it is secreted by the placenta
(C) its plasma level is low during the menses
(D) its plasma level remains constant after implantation
(E) its plasma level rises subsequent to ovulation

430. The anti-inflammatory effect of cortisol treatment is thought to be due to all the following mechanisms EXCEPT

(A) decreased capillary membrane permeability
(B) decreased formation of leukotrienes
(C) increased release of pyrogen from granulocytes
(D) inhibition of phospholipase A_2
(E) stabilization of cellular lysosomal membranes

431. In women, estrogens have all the following effects EXCEPT

(A) they facilitate the growth of ovarian follicles
(B) they cause cyclic changes in the vagina and endometrium
(C) they cause cervical mucus to become thinner and more alkaline
(D) they produce ductal proliferation in the breast
(E) they produce glandular proliferation in the breast

432. Cholesterol is the precursor in the adrenal biosynthesis of all the following compounds EXCEPT

(A) aldosterone
(B) cortisol
(C) dexamethasone
(D) testosterone
(E) estradiol

433. Thyroid-stimulating hormone (TSH) increases circulating thyroid hormone levels by increasing all the following EXCEPT

(A) thyroid-binding protein concentrations
(B) proteolysis of thyroglobulin in the follicles
(C) activity of the iodide pump
(D) size of thyroid cells
(E) number of thyroid cells

434. Testosterone is synthesized from all the following substances EXCEPT

(A) androstenedione
(B) cholesterol
(C) dehydroepiandrosterone
(D) estrogen
(E) pregnenolone

435. Glucagon characteristically increases all the following EXCEPT

(A) gluconeogenesis in the liver
(B) glycogenolysis in the liver
(C) glycogenolysis in muscle
(D) ketogenesis in the liver
(E) lipolysis in adipose tissue

436. Male hypogonadism could be produced by a lesion in all the following sites EXCEPT the

(A) testes
(B) pituitary gland
(C) pineal gland
(D) hypothalamus
(E) globus pallidus

DIRECTIONS: Each group of questions below consists of lettered headings followed by a set of numbered items. For each numbered item select the **one** lettered heading with which it is **most** closely associated. Each lettered heading may be used **once, more than once, or not at all.**

Questions 437–443

For each hormone listed below, select the statement that best describes its mechanism of action.

(A) Binds to cell surface receptors and stimulates production of cyclic nucleotides in the cytoplasm
(B) Interacts with a cytoplasmic receptor, then localizes in the nucleus and directs protein and nucleotide synthesis
(C) Binds to cell surface receptors and then activates intracellular processes by a mediator other than cyclic nucleotides
(D) Interacts with a cytoplasmic receptor, then localizes in mitochondria and directs oxidative metabolism
(E) None of the above

437. 1,25-Dihydroxycholecalciferol

438. Thyrotropin-releasing hormone

439. Epinephrine

440. Insulin

441. Luteinizing hormone

442. Cortisol

443. Thyroxine

Questions 444–447

For each hormone that follows, select its appropriate function in breast development and lactation.

(A) Plays a background role in breast development
(B) Stimulates development of alveolar components
(C) Stimulates growth of ductal system
(D) Stimulates milk let-down
(E) None of the above

444. Progesterone

445. Estradiol

446. Oxytocin

447. Insulin

Questions 448–450

For each situation described below, select the lettered curve on the graph that best represents the blood glucose pattern of the animal in question.

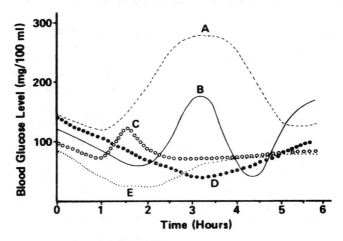

448. A normal dog receives an intravenous injection of pure crystalline insulin without glucose at time zero

449. An alloxan-treated diabetic dog goes without food for 12 h and is given a glucose meal at time 1 h

450. A normal dog goes without food for 12 h and is given glucose at time 1 h

Questions 451–455

For each of the hormones listed below, select the pancreatic islet cell by which it is secreted.

(A)   A (α) cell
(B)   B (β) cell
(C)   D (δ) cell
(D)   F cell
(E)   None of the above

451. Somatostatin

452. Secretin

453. Insulin

454. Glucagon

455. Pancreatic polypeptide

Endocrine Physiology
Answers

371. The answer is A. *(Guyton, 8/e, pp 827–828.)* It is thought that the secretion of antidiuretic hormone (ADH)—also called *arginine vasopressin (AVP)*—and oxytocin by the neurohypophysis is regulated in the hypothalamic supraoptic and paraventricular nuclei, respectively. This hypothalamic control of secretion of pituitary hormone (inhibitory as well as releasing) in the case of the neurohypophysis is by direct neural connection, and in the case of the adenohypophysis by humoral factors conveyed by a microcirculation known as the *hypothalamic-hypophyseal portal system.*

372. The answer is E. *(Ganong, 16/e, pp 355–357.)* PTH, secreted by the chief cells of the parathyroid gland, is essential for life. The secretion of PTH is inversely related to the circulating levels of ionized calcium. PTH has a direct effect on bone involving cAMP changes in osteoblast and osteocyte permeability. It also increases calcium absorption from the gut, although that effect is the result of PTH-mediated increases in renal 1,2,5-dihydroxycholecalciferol.

373. The answer is C. *(Berne, 3/e, pp 846–848.)* Fasting persons are characterized by decreases in endogenous stores of carbohydrates, fats, and proteins and are said to be in a state of catabolism. As an adaptation, BMR decreases to limit the drain on energy stores. Catabolism of muscle protein is reflected in a rising excretion of nitrogen in the urine. Although glucose is an essential fuel for the central nervous system, with prolonged fasting two-thirds of the energy needs are met by ketoacids. As long as sufficient fluids are ingested, a healthy person can survive up to 60 days.

374. The answer is E. *(Berne, 3/e, pp 770–776.)* ANH is a polypeptide hormone produced in the atria from preatriopeptigen, which increases salt and water excretion by the kidneys. ANH is secreted in response to a variety of stimuli including atrial distention due to hypervolemia. Vasodilation of the afferent and efferent arterioles of the glomerulus increases GFR. This effect combined with inhibition of aldosterone and renin secretion promotes natriuresis and diuresis.

375. The answer is B. *(Berne, 3/e, pp 990–996.)* Throughout the reproductive life of the human male, 100 to 200 million sperm are produced daily. Of critical importance to the hormonal regulation of spermatogenesis is the pulsatile release of GRH and the subsequent involvement of FSH and LH at their target cells. FSH acts directly on the Sertoli cells of the seminiferous tubules to initiate mitotic and meiotic activity of germ cells. LH effects are thought to be mediated via stimulation of testosterone secretion by the Leydig cells.

376. The answer is B. *(Berne, 3/e, pp 914–920. Johnson, pp 659–662.)* Growth hormone (GH), also known as *somatotropin*, is among a group of tropic hormones, including prolactin, ACTH, TSH, LH, and FSH, that are synthesized, stored, and secreted by the endocrine cells of the anterior pituitary. Its release is stimulated by growth hormone–releasing hormone and inhibited by somatostatin. Numerous factors serve as a stimulus for GH release, including hypoglycemia (e.g., insulin administration); moderate to severe exercise; stress due to emotional disturbances, illness, and fever; and dopamine agonists such as bromocriptine.

377. The answer is C. *(Berne, 3/e, pp 689–696. Johnson, pp 1003–1006.)* The menstrual cycle is divided physiologically into three phases. The follicular phase begins with the onset of menstrual bleeding and ranges in duration from 9 to 23 days. The ovulatory phase lasts 1 to 3 days and culminates in ovulation. The luteal phase, the most constant phase of the menstrual cycle, lasts about 14 days and ends with the onset of menstrual bleeding. In a woman with a menstrual cycle of 28 to 30 days, ovulation would be expected to occur between days 14 and 16.

378. The answer is B. *(Berne, 3/e, pp 897–902. Johnson, pp 551–558.)* The pituitary gland (the hypophysis) is located just beneath the hypothalamus and is connected to the hypothalamus by the infundibulum. It is a compound gland consisting of an anterior lobe (adenohypophysis) and a neural, or posterior, lobe. The anterior pituitary secretes six physiologically important hormones that govern the function of the thyroid (TSH) and adrenal glands (ACTH), the mammary glands (prolactin), and the gonads (FSH, LH) as well as regulate growth (GH). Oxytocin is secreted by the posterior pituitary and is involved in lactation and parturition.

379. The answer is D. *(Berne, 3/e, pp 920–923.)* Prolactin is a single-chain protein secreted by the anterior pituitary whose principal physiologic effects involve breast development and milk production. Consistent with its role in lactogenesis, prolactin secretion increases during pregnancy. Unique among the pituitary hormones, prolactin secretion is tonically inhibited by the hypothalamus. Dopamine has many characteristics of the hypothalamic inhibitory factor, although it is not found in the hypothalamus.

380. The answer is C. *(Ganong, 16/e, pp 323–324. West, 12/e, p 828.)* During fetal life, the adrenal cortex consists of a thin subcapsular rim, which eventually gives rise to the adult cortex, and a thick inner fetal cortex, which constitutes 80 percent of the gland. This zone undergoes rapid involution after birth. Because it lacks 3β-hydroxysteroid dehydrogenase, the enzyme that converts pregnenolone to progesterone (the initial step in both glucocorticoid and mineralocorticoid synthesis), the fetal cortex synthesizes primarily dehydroepiandrosterone. This steroid is released as its sulfate and is metabolized further to estrogen and androgen by the placenta.

381. The answer is B. *(Guyton, 8/e, pp 746, 857–858.)* Glucose will not diffuse through a cell membrane against a concentration gradient; in many cells diffusion is facilitated in the presence of insulin. Such transport is enhanced, for example, in skeletal, cardiac, some smooth muscle, and adipose tissue. Insulin does not enhance glucose transport into brain cells, through intestinal mucosa, or through tubular epithelium of the kidney.

382. The answer is B. *(Ganong, 16/e, pp 264–265.)* At rest, the caloric needs of skeletal muscle are met primarily by mitochondrial oxidation of free fatty acids derived from adipose tissue. Glucose is used primarily by the brain and erythrocytes. During prolonged exercise, skeletal muscle becomes relatively anaerobic when compared with its resting state and relies heavily upon glycolysis for ATP production. The increase in glucose required is met primarily by glycogenolysis and gluconeogenesis in the liver. Gluconeogenesis does not occur in skeletal muscle. Thus, long-distance runners "carbohydrate load" before a race to increase hepatic glycogen stores. Intestinal uptake of glucose is influenced primarily by dietary intake, which would not ordinarily increase during exercise.

383. The answer is B. *(Ganong, 16/e, pp 341–343.)* Aldosterone acts upon epithelial cells of the nephrons, sweat glands, salivary glands, and the gastrointestinal tract to promote the conservation of sodium and the excretion of potassium. As a consequence of sodium retention, there is a modest expansion of extracellular fluid volume and thus an increase in body weight. With expansion of extracellular volume, blood pressure also increases.

384. The answer is D. *(Ganong, 16/e, pp 330, 341, 392.)* Cortisol is the only hormone that has a diurnal variation, as shown in the graph accompanying the question. Plasma cortisol levels rise sharply during sleep, peaking soon after awakening, and sinking to a low level approximately 12 h later. This pattern is intimately related to the secretory rhythm of ACTH, which governs — and in turn is partly governed by — plasma concentration of cortisol.

385. The answer is C. *(Guyton, 8/e, pp 899–903.)* Ovulation takes place just after the peak of the luteinizing hormone (LH) and estrogen curves, which occurs on approximately the fourteenth day of the menstrual cycle. Although FSH is primarily responsible for follicular maturation within the ovary, LH is necessary for final follicular maturation; without it, ovulation cannot take place. Both estrogen, following a sharp preovulatory rise in plasma concentration, and progesterone are secreted in abundance by the postovulatory corpus luteum.

386. The answer is B. *(Guyton, 8/e, pp 831–833.)* The thyroid gland has a specialized active transport system that very efficiently traps iodide from circulating blood and can accumulate iodide against a large concentration gradient. Within the thyroid, the iodide rapidly undergoes organification by which it is oxidized and covalently linked to tyrosine residues in thyroglobulin. Thus, it is in thyroglobulin that iodide is principally stored within the thyroid gland. The iodinated tyrosine residues gradually become coupled to form thyroxine, the major secretion product of the thyroid.

387. The answer is D. *(Ganong, 16/e, pp 395–400.)* There is a marked increase in progesterone secretion following ovulation. Almost all the progesterone secreted in nonpregnant women is secreted by the corpus luteum. Secretion of both progesterone and estrogen is controlled by luteinizing hormone (LH) released by the adenohypophysis, and LH release itself is under the direction of a hypothalamic releasing factor.

388. The answer is B. *(Guyton, 8/e, pp 831–833.)* Thyroxine is the main thyroid hormone entering the circulation and constitutes approximately 95 percent of active plasma thyroid hormone; the percentage remaining is almost entirely triiodothyronine, which, although more potent than thyroxine, has a more transient presence. Thyroglobulin is the principal storage form of thyroid hormone within the gland and very little is released into the blood. Thyrotropin (TSH) and long-acting thyroid stimulator (LATS) both stimulate thyroid hormone production and growth of the thyroid gland.

389. The answer is E. *(Guyton, 8/e, p 833.)* Circulating thyroxine can be bound to albumin, thyroxine-binding prealbumin (TBPA), or thyroxine-binding globulin (TBG). Most thyroxine is bound, and despite the large available pool of albumin, most of it is bound to TBG. This reflects the relatively greater affinity of TBG for thyroxine. Only the free unbound form of thyroxine is physiologically active.

390. The answer is C. *(Berne, 3/e, pp 1006–1009. Ganong, 16/e, pp 361–363.)* Preparation of primordial ovarian follicles for ovulation is the primary function of follicle-stimulating hormone (FSH). During the initial 10 to 14 days of the menstrual cycle, secretion of FSH stimulates development of the theca and granulosa cells of the follicle and promotes their synthesis of estrogens, including estradiol. When estrogen reaches a certain level, a sudden surge of secretion of FSH and luteinizing hormone (LH) occurs, followed by ovulation. The surge in LH then promotes luteinization of the postovulatory follicle and stimulates the production of progesterone by the resultant corpus luteum. If pregnancy occurs, chorionic gonadotropin (hCG) is secreted by the placenta and replaces the stimulation of production of progesterone by LH.

391. The answer is E. *(Guyton, 8/e, pp 907–908.)* In response to estrogen secretion by the ovary, the endometrial lining of the uterus undergoes proliferation of both glandular epithelium and supporting stroma during the first 10 to 14 days of the menstrual cycle. Following ovulation (point A on the graph accompanying the question) the glands begin to secrete mucus and the stroma undergoes pseudodecidual reaction in preparation for potential pregnancy. When ovulation is not followed by implantation of a fertilized ovum, progesterone secretion declines as the corpus luteum involutes, and the endometrial lining is almost completely shed during menses.

392. The answer is A. *(Guyton, 8/e, pp 919–920.)* Human chorionic gonadotropin (hCG) begins to appear in the maternal blood approximately 6 to 8 days following ovulation, upon implantation of the fertilized ovum in the endometrium. The secretion of hCG is essential to prevent involution of the corpus luteum and to stimulate secretion of progesterone and estrogens, which continues until the placenta becomes large enough to secrete sufficient quantities of those hormones. Following a peak at 7 to 9 weeks, hCG secretion gradually declines to a low level by 20 weeks gestation.

393. The answer is A. *(West, 12/e, pp 761–763.)* Most, if not all, of the effects of insulin begin with the binding of insulin to its specific membrane receptor. This binding is associated with autophosphorylation of tyrosine residues in the receptor molecule and exhibits "negative cooperativity"; that is, binding of one molecule of insulin reduces the affinity of the receptor for a second molecule of insulin that would completely saturate its binding sites. Prolonged elevation of plasma insulin levels leads to a reduction in the number of available receptor molecules ("down-regulation") so that the effect of a given dose of insulin is diminished. Insulin-receptor binding is required for initiation of the effects of insulin on the enhanced transport of glucose, amino acids, and potassium into cells.

394. The answer is B. *(Ganong, 16/e, p 278. West, 12/e, pp 744–746.)* Hormone-sensitive lipase is a cytoplasmic enzyme in adipocytes that catalyzes the complete hydrolysis of triglyceride to fatty acids and glycerol. It is activated by a cyclic AMP–dependent protein kinase that phosphorylates the enzyme, converting it to its active form. Since no accumulation of monoglycerides or diglycerides is detected in adipocytes following the action of hormone-sensitive lipase, it is the initial hydrolysis of triglyceride to fatty acid and diglyceride that is the rate-limiting step. Hormone-sensitive lipase is sensitive to several hormones in vitro, but it appears to be regulated in vivo primarily by epinephrine and glucagon, which activate it by increasing cyclic AMP, and insulin, which inhibits it by preventing cyclic AMP–dependent phosphorylation. Cortisol enhances lipolysis indirectly by promoting increased enzyme synthesis.

395. The answer is D. *(Berne, 3/e, pp 990–996. West, 12/e, pp 851–853, 858–859.)* Spermatogenesis occurs within the seminiferous tubules of the testis and requires secretion of both FSH and LH. FSH acts directly on the seminiferous tubules while the effects of LH are thought to be due to its stimulation of secretion of testosterone by the Leydig cells. Spermatogonia are the stem cells, which divide several times by mitosis to produce more stem cells and type B spermatogonia. The type B spermatogonia give rise to primary spermatocytes, which undergo meiosis. Normally, 100 to 200 million sperm are produced per day. Complete maturation of spermatozoa within the seminiferous tubules requires approximately 70 days in man.

396. The answer is C. *(West, 12/e, pp 851, 856, 858–859.)* The Sertoli cells rest on a basal lamina and form a layer around the periphery of the seminiferous tubules. They are attached to each other by specialized junctional complexes that limit the movement of fluid and solute molecules from the interstitial space and blood to the tubular lumen and thus form a blood-testis barrier that provides an immunologically privileged environment for sperm maturation. Sertoli cells are intimately associated with developing spermatozoa and play a major role in germ-cell maturation. They secrete a variety of serum proteins and an androgen-binding protein into the tubular fluid in response to FSH and testosterone stimulation. Testosterone is synthesized and secreted by the interstitial Leydig cells. Estrogen is produced in small amounts by the Sertoli cells before puberty.

397. The answer is C. *(Ganong, 16/e, pp 436–437.)* Iron is transported in the blood plasma bound to the beta globulin transferrin. Excess iron is stored in all cells, but especially in liver cells, combined with the protein apoferritin; the storage complex of iron plus protein is called *ferritin*. The rate of iron absorption is extremely slow, with a maximal rate of only a few milligrams per day. Iron absorption is an active process. Because iron is absorbed mainly in the ferrous rather than ferric form, ferrous iron compounds are more effective in treating iron deficiency than are ferric compounds.

398. The answer is E. *(Ganong, 16/e, p 302.)* The islets of Langerhans, which constitute 1 to 2 percent of the weight of the pancreas, contain at least four types of cells: A (α), B (β), D (δ), and F cells. The A cells secrete glucagon, the B cells secrete insulin, the D cells secrete somatostatin, and the F cells secrete pancreatic polypeptide. There are more islets in the tail than in the head or body of the pancreas, and each islet has a copious blood supply.

399. The answer is D. *(Ganong, 16/e, pp 355–357.)* The main function of the parathyroid gland is to maintain a constant ionized calcium level in the extracellular fluid. To do this, parathyroid hormone stimulates increased plasma calcium levels, chiefly by mobilizing calcium from bones. Although parathyroid hormone can also increase renal tubular reabsorption of calcium and intestinal absorption of calcium, these effects depend on adequate dietary ingestion of calcium and thus occur more slowly.

400. The answer is A. *(Ganong, 16/e, pp 357–359.)* Parathyroid hormone is essential for maintaining normal plasma calcium and phosphate concentrations. Parathyroid hormone is released in response to low plasma calcium concentrations and acts to increase phosphate excretion and calcium reabsorption. If parathyroid hormone concentrations rise above normal levels, plasma calcium concentrations will increase and plasma concentrations of phosphate will decrease. Calcitonin is released by the thyroid gland when plasma concentrations of calcium increase. Thus the increase in calcium associated with hyperparathyroidism will cause an increase in the secretion of calcitonin. Sodium and potassium levels are not affected by a decrease in parathyroid hormone levels.

401. The answer is B. *(Berne, 3/e, pp 914–920.)* Human growth hormone (GH) is a peptide that is synthesized and released from the anterior pituitary. Its release is stimulated by growth hormone–releasing hormone (GHRH) and inhibited by somatostatin. Both of these peptides are synthesized and released by the hypothalamus and their releases are regulated by multiple feedback loops. GH has the direct effect on adipose tissue of decreasing glucose uptake and increasing lipolysis. It also acts to increase the production and release of somatomedins from the liver. These peptides have a multitude of effects on the body and promote growth of organs, bones, and lean body mass.

402. The answer is D. *(Guyton, 8/e, pp 822–824.)* Growth hormone exerts a wide variety of effects on body metabolism, including increased protein synthesis, decreased use of carbohydrate, and increased use of fat. The net effect of the hormone's action is the accumulation of protein and conservation of carbohydrate at the expense of fat stores. In addition to those effects, growth hormone promotes growth by stimulating synthesis of cartilage and bone via the actions of somatomedin C (insulin-like growth factor 1 [IGF-1]).

403. The answer is C. *(Ganong, 16/e, pp 316–318. Guyton, 8/e, pp 862–863.)* The primary action of glucagon is to increase blood glucose concentration, which it accomplishes by promoting gluconeogenesis and glycogenolysis in the liver but not in muscle. These effects are mediated by cyclic AMP, which is produced by hepatic adenyl cyclase following interaction of glucagon with its plasma membrane receptor. Interaction of glucagon with different hepatic plasma membrane receptors activates phospholipase C, which results in a rise in concentration of intracellular Ca^{2+}, which further stimulates glycogenolysis. Although glucagon opposes the action of insulin, it does not directly affect insulin secretion.

404. The answer is D. *(Ganong, 16/e, pp 297–298.)* The major action of parathyroid hormone is to increase plasma calcium concentration by mobilization of calcium from bones, increasing absorption of calcium by the intestine, and decreasing the secretion of calcium by the kidney. When a person is unable to secrete a normal amount of parathyroid hormone, calcium levels fall, which leads to tetany, a condition in which the excitability of nerves and muscles increases. The increase in excitability results from a lowering of the voltage at which an action potential can be elicited. Threshold can be reduced so low that tapping a muscle can cause it to contract.

405. The answer is A. *(Ganong, 16/e, pp 408–411.)* During early pregnancy, human chorionic gonadotropin (hCG) secretion increases steadily, reaching a peak at 8 to 9 weeks following implantation of the fertilized ovum. Estriol and pregnanediol—estrogen and progesterone metabolites—are excreted in the urine. Their excretion and that of human chorionic somatomammotropin (hCS), a peptide hormone similar to human growth hormone, increase steadily and peak just before parturition. Oxytocin is important in the development of uterine contractions during labor and is secreted in the greatest amounts only at parturition, when uterine sensitivity to the hormone is maximal.

406. The answer is A. *(Ganong, 16/e, pp 303–305.)* Proinsulin, a single-chain polypeptide, is a precursor of insulin. The insulin molecule is composed of two polypeptide chains, which are linked via disulfide bonds. In proinsulin these two chains are linked by an intervening peptide sequence termed *C (con-*

necting) peptide. Cleavage of proinsulin to insulin and C peptide takes place in the Golgi complex so that equimolar amounts of insulin and C peptide are secreted by the β cell. Proinsulin shows some immunologic cross-reactivity with insulin but is much less biologically active.

407. The answer is D. *(Ganong, 16/e, pp 305–308.)* One of insulin's major effects is the stimulation of the Na-K pump, which increases potassium entry into cells. Insulin given along with glucose, to prevent hypoglycemia, is often used as a treatment for hyperkalemia. Insulin's major effect on metabolism is the synthesis of proteins and lipids and the storage of glucose as glycogen. Insulin stimulates the uptake of amino acids and glucose by most cells of the body and decreases the rate of gluconeogenesis. Insulin has no effect on urine formation, but in diabetes, when glucose levels increase to a level at which the kidney can no longer reabsorb the filtered glucose, glucose acts as an osmotic diuretic and increases the formation of urine.

408. The answer is A. *(Ganong, 16/e, pp 338–344.)* The secretion of ACTH occurs in several irregular bursts during the day; the peak occurs early in the morning prior to awakening and thus is not due to the stress of arising. This circadian rhythm—maximum secretion in early morning, minimum in the evening—is regulated by the hypothalamus through the secretion of corticotropin-releasing hormone (CRH) into the hypothalamic-hypophyseal portal capillary system. In addition to the basal rhythm, physical or mental stress will lead to increased ACTH secretion within minutes. ACTH is also regulated as a result of feedback inhibition by the hormones whose synthesis it stimulates, e.g., glucocorticoids. Aldosterone is a mineralocorticoid and not controlled by ACTH. Epinephrine does not appear to have any effect on ACTH secretion.

409. The answer is E. *(Berne, 3/e, pp 942–944.)* Thyroid hormone affects all aspects of metabolism; it increases calorigenesis in every tissue in the body. The hormone stimulates protein synthesis, which may be directly responsible for a portion of its calorigenic effect. Thyroid hormone affects both synthesis and degradation of lipids; the net effect is a decrease in lipid stores. By increasing the mechanisms by which cholesterol is eliminated from the body, thyroid hormone decreases plasma cholesterol levels. Because of its stimulatory effect on metabolic processes, thyroid hormone increases the demand for coenzymes and vitamins.

410. The answer is B. *(Ganong, 16/e, pp 342–345.)* The symptoms of primary hyperaldosteronism (Conn's syndrome) develop from chronic excess secretion of aldosterone from the zona glomerulosa of the adrenal cortex. Patients are hypertensive and have an expanded volume with a decreased hematocrit. They are not markedly hypernatremic because of a renal escape phenomenon. Patients are severely depleted of potassium and as a consequence suffer kidney damage, with a resulting loss in concentrating ability.

411. The answer is A. *(Berne, 3/e, pp 949–954, 971–976.)* The adrenal glands are complex, multifunctional endocrine organs essential for life. The adrenal cortex, the outer layer of the adrenal gland, secretes steroid hormones that are derivatives of cholesterol. They include the mineralocorticoid aldosterone; the glucocorticoids cortisol and corticosterone; and androstenedione, the sex steroid hormone. Epinephrine is the principal secretion of the inner zone of the adrenal gland, the medulla.

412. The answer is A. *(Guyton, 8/e, p 852.)* Removal of the adrenal glands produces the clinical picture known as Addison's disease, a disorder associated with deprivation of adrenocortical hormones. Thus, a lack of glucocorticoids diminishes the body's ability to synthesize glucose by gluconeogenesis. Severe mineralocorticoid deprivation produces grave fluid and electrolyte disturbances as an ultimate consequence of impaired sodium reabsorption, excessive potassium plasma levels, and acidosis.

413. The answer is E. *(Ganong, 16/e, pp 355–357.)* An increase of parathyroid hormone (PTH) in the body causes an increase in the level of plasma calcium by mobilizing calcium from bones and by increasing reabsorption of calcium in the kidneys. It also increases intestinal absorption of calcium by increasing formation of 1,25-dihydroxycholecalciferol. PTH causes a decrease in the level of plasma phosphate by decreasing renal proximal tubular reabsorption of phosphate. Despite increased renal reabsorption of calcium, hypercalciuria occurs and kidney stones containing calcium are commonly formed during hyperparathyroidism because the increased amount of calcium filtered exceeds the renal reabsorptive capacity.

414. The answer is D. *(Guyton, 8/e, pp 746, 857–858.)* Insulin increases glucose uptake in skeletal muscle, cardiac muscle, smooth muscle, adipose tissue, leukocytes, and the liver. It does not do so in the brain (except probably in part of the hypothalamus), renal tubules, intestinal mucosa, or red blood cells. In most insulin-sensitive tissues, insulin acts to promote glucose transport by enhancing facilitated diffusion of glucose down a concentration gradient. In the liver, where glucose freely permeates the cell membrane, glucose uptake is increased as a result of its phosphorylation by glucokinase. Formation of glucose-6-phosphate reduces the intracellular concentration of free glucose and maintains the concentration gradient favoring movement of glucose into the cell.

415. The answer is E. *(Guyton, 8/e, pp 746–747, 835.)* Epinephrine and glucagon stimulate glycogenolysis in the liver by means of a mechanism dependent on cyclic adenosine monophosphate. Thyroxine, glucagon, and ACTH (by increasing cortisol secretion) also enhance gluconeogenesis from amino acid precursors. Both of these processes result in hyperglycemia. Aldosterone, a mineralocorticoid involved in sodium regulation, has no direct effect on glucose metabolism.

416. The answer is B. *(Ganong, 16/e, pp 414–416. Guyton, 8/e, pp 211–215.)* Angiotensin II is an octapeptide produced in response to hypovolemia by the combined action of renin, released from the juxtaglomerular apparatus, and angiotensin-converting enzyme in the lung. It has a number of actions, all of which are directed toward increasing arterial pressure. The actions include (1) direct vasoconstriction of peripheral arterioles; (2) stimulation of aldosterone secretion by the adrenal cortex, resulting in increased sodium tubular resorption; and (3) stimulation of the subfornical organ of the diencephalon, which activates neural areas concerned with thirst. The latter two actions, by increasing blood volume, play a role in long-term regulation of blood pressure. Angiotensin II also exerts negative feedback on its own production by inhibiting renin secretion. It does not act directly on renal tubules to influence salt excretion.

417. The answer is C. *(Berne, 3/e, pp 942–947.)* Hypothyroidism is a condition usually characterized by low levels of T_3 and T_4 owing to atrophy of the thyroid gland. In very rare cases there is resistance to the effects of thyroid hormones. A deficiency of thyroid hormones or their effects results in bradycardia, which is due to decreased sympathetic activity, and a decreased metabolic rate with its associated sleepiness, weight gain, and cold intolerance. Excess thyroid hormones increase metabolic rate, which increases heat production, stimulates the appetite, and causes weight loss even in the face of increased intake of food. Heat intolerance is characteristic of hyperthyroidism.

418. The answer is D. *(Ganong, 16/e, pp 296–300.)* Goiter, or thyroid enlargement, can occur in association with any level of thyroid function. Thyroid growth is controlled primarily by thyroid-stimulating hormone (TSH). Increased levels of TSH could occur with a pituitary adenoma or as a consequence of diminished negative feedback by thyroid hormone on the hypothalamus owing to decreased synthesis of the hormone. A decrease in synthesis of thyroid hormone would accompany iodine deficiency or ingestion of goitrogens, which inhibit iodination reactions in the thyroid. Goitrogens may be found in cabbage or turnips. In Graves' disease, an immunoglobulin that binds to TSH receptors causes an increase in thyroid size. Excessive intake of thyroxine would suppress TSH secretion and not cause thyroid enlargement.

419. The answer is C. *(Ganong, 16/e, pp 364–370, 386.)* Synthesis and secretion of growth hormone by the anterior pituitary is regulated by a variety of metabolic factors, many of which act to alter the balance between release of growth hormone–releasing hormone (GRH) and somatostatin (SS) from the hypothalamus. Insulin-induced hypoglycemia is a major stimulus for release of growth hormone. Amino acids are also potent stimuli for release of growth hormone, while fatty acids are inhibitory. Deep sleep induces the greatest daily peak in secretion of growth hormone. Thyroxine acts directly on pituitary cells to enhance synthesis of growth hormone and is required for the normal responsiveness of the pituitary and hypothalamus to physiologic stimuli.

420. The answer is A. *(Ganong, 16/e, pp 253–256.)* The basal metabolic rate (BMR) is the metabolic rate measured at rest 12 to 14 h after a meal. It is influenced by a number of factors and correlates well with body surface area. Increases in epinephrine secretion, which occur in an anxious person even at rest, increase metabolic rate. Environmental temperature also influences BMR. At low temperatures (e.g., 20°C) heat-conserving mechanisms are activated and BMR rises. At elevated environmental temperatures (e.g., 35 to 40°C) when body temperature also rises slightly, BMR again rises. BMR is high in children and decreases with advancing age.

421. The answer is E. *(West, 12/e, pp 746–747.)* The uptake of triglycerides into adipose tissue and other tissues from plasma lipoproteins requires hydrolysis of triglyceride to fatty acids and glycerol by an enzyme bound to the endothelial surface, lipoprotein lipase. The activity of this enzyme varies in reciprocal fashion with that of cytoplasmic hormone-sensitive lipase; e.g., its activity is enhanced by insulin and glucose and decreased by catecholamines. Lipoprotein lipase is present in nearly every tissue and acts at the capillary surface as it does in adipose tissue. Receptor-mediated endocytosis is important in the turnover of the protein portion of plasma lipoproteins.

422. The answer is D. *(Ganong, 16/e, pp 395–398, 408–413.)* Fertilization and early cleavage of the zygote occur in the fallopian tube in the human female. After approximately 3 days, the zygote enters the uterine cavity, where it undergoes additional divisions over a period of 3 to 4 days to form a morula of approximately 60 cells that is transformed into a blastocyst consisting of the yolk sac and embryo. Enzymatic digestion of the zona pellucida and infiltration of the endometrium by the syncytiotrophoblast, which forms the outer layer of the blastocyst, result in implantation of the blastocyst within the endometrium, where it erodes into maternal vessels. During these early stages of embryogenesis, the endometrium is primed by progesterone secreted by the corpus luteum in the ovary in response to pituitary gonadotropin secretion. After 10 to 15 days, placental gonadotropins maintain the corpus luteum until placental synthesis of progesterone is established at 6 to 8 weeks of gestation.

423. The answer is D. *(Ganong, 16/e, p 332.)* Inappropriate virilization manifested by frontal balding and increased facial hair in a female could be a result of excessive amounts of exogenous or endogenous androgens. Small amounts of androgens are normally produced in the female by the adrenal glands and ovaries. Thus, tumors of either the adrenal or ovary might be associated with virilization. Deficiency of 11β-hydroxylase, by leading to hypersecretion of 11-deoxycortisol and 11-deoxycorticosterone, a weak mineralocorticoid, results in a diversion of steroid precursors to androgen-synthesizing pathways. A patient thus affected would manifest both virilization and hypertension.

424. The answer is D. *(Ganong, 16/e, pp 290–293.)* Less than 0.2 percent of plasma triiodothyronine and thyroxine circulate as the free molecule. The three major proteins that bind these hormones in the blood are (1) thyroxine-binding globulin (TBG), (2) thyroxine-binding prealbumin (TBPA), and (3) albumin. Of the three, albumin has the greatest capacity for hormone binding, but its affinity for thyroid hormone is relatively low. Consequently, most of the triiodothyronine and thyroxine circulate bound to TBG and TBPA. Only the free form of the hormone is physiologically active. Thyroglobulin is the form in which the thyroid hormones are stored within the thyroid.

425. The answer is B. *(Guyton, 8/e, pp 831–835.)* Thyroglobulin, the storage form of thyroid hormones, is stored extracellularly in follicles lined by thyroid epithelium. Only about 0.02 percent of the thyroxine and about 0.2 percent of the triiodothyronine are normally present in plasma in the free form; the rest is bound to thyroxine-binding globulin, thyroxine-binding prealbumin, and albumin. Following injection of thyroxine into a human, the effect on the metabolic rate is not noticeable for 2 to 3 days; then the rate begins to increase progressively and reaches a maximum in 10 to 12 days. Some of the activity persists for up to 2 months. The principal effect of the thyroid hormones is an increase in the metabolic rate of most tissues in the body, with a few exceptions such as brain, retina, testes, spleen, and lungs.

426. The answer is B. *(Ganong, 16/e, pp 422–423.)* Melatonin is synthesized in the pineal gland from the amino acid tryptophan. Synthesis and secretion of melatonin are increased in the dark via input from norepinephrine secreted by postganglionic sympathetic neurons. Pinealomas (tumors of the pineal gland) that destroy the pineal gland, reduce secretion of melatonin, and cause hypothalamic damage may cause precocious puberty by removing the inhibitory effect of melatonin on the pituitary response to gonadotropin-releasing hormone. Melatonin causes amphibian skin to become lighter in color but has no role in the regulation of skin color in humans.

427. The answer is E. *(Guyton, 8/e, pp 855–860.)* α-Glycerophosphate is produced in the course of normal use of glucose. In the absence of adequate quantities of α-glycerophosphate—a normal acceptor of free fatty acids in triglyceride synthesis—lipolysis will be the predominant process in adipose tissue. As a result, fatty acids will be released into the blood. The prevailing insulin level is decisive in the selection of substrate by a tissue for the production of energy. Insulin promotes use of carbohydrate, and a lack of the hormone causes use of fat mainly to the exclusion of uptake and use of glucose, except by brain tissue. Indirect depression of use of glucose by excess fatty acids is a result, and not a contributing cause, of increased use of fat.

428. The answer is D. *(Ganong, 16/e, pp 313–316.)* Blood glucose levels affect the pancreatic islets directly and constitute the major control mechanism of insulin secretion; adequate quantities of Ca^{2+} and K^+ are also required for normal secretion. 2-Deoxyglucose, a nonmetabolized analogue of glucose, inhibits insulin secretion, as does somatostatin, a polypeptide present in the D (δ) cells of the pancreatic islets (and in several other tissues). Thiazide diuretics, not an osmotic diuretic such as the inert sugar mannitol, inhibit insulin secretion in some patients.

429. The answer is D. *(Berne, 3/e, pp 1009–1012, 1016–1017.)* The plasma level of progesterone is low during the menses and remains low until just prior to ovulation. It rises substantially after ovulation owing to secretion by the corpus luteum. If fertilization occurs, the corpus luteum continues to secrete progesterone until the placenta develops and begins to produce large amounts of the hormone. The plasma level of progesterone rises steadily throughout pregnancy after the placenta takes over production at about 12 weeks of gestation.

430. The answer is C. *(Ganong, 16/e, pp 332–333.)* The anti-inflammatory effects of exogenous cortisol are due to its ability to decrease capillary membrane permeability and probably also to its ability to stabilize lysosomal membranes and decrease the formation of bradykinin. Glucocorticoids inhibit the enzyme phospholipase A_2. This decreases the release of arachidonic acid and the variety of substances produced from it, such as leukotrienes, prostaglandins, thromboxanes, and prostacyclin. Cortisol owes its fever-reducing action to the hormone's ability to decrease the release of pyrogen (interleukin 1) from granulocytes. However, only in massive doses will the hormone achieve the effects described. Endogenous cortisol does not exert significant anti-inflammatory action.

431. The answer is E. *(Ganong, 16/e, pp 400–403.)* Estrogens can stimulate growth of ovarian follicles even in hypophysectomized women. Estrogens also stimulate growth of the glandular epithelium of the endometrium, the smooth muscle of the uterus, and the uterine vascular system. The epithelium of the vagina is so sensitive to estrogen action that vaginal smear examination is used for a bioassay of the hormone. Estrogens cause the mucus secreted by the cervix to become thinner and more alkaline and to exhibit a fernlike pattern upon drying. Growth of the *glandular* elements of the breast is stimulated by progesterone; growth of the *ductal* elements is stimulated by estrogen.

432. The answer is C. *(Ganong, 16/e, pp 328–331.)* Cholesterol is the precursor for biosynthesis of all adrenal steroids. The rate-limiting step in their biosynthesis is conversion of cholesterol to pregnenolone by stepwise hydroxylation. From that point, divergent pathways result in synthesis of glucocorticoids (cortisol and corticosterone), mineralocorticoids (aldosterone), and small amounts of estrogen (estradiol) and androgen (testosterone). Dexamethasone is a synthetic steroid with potent glucocorticoid activity.

433. The answer is A. *(Ganong, 16/e, pp 296–297.)* Thyroid-stimulating hormone (TSH) increases all metabolic activities of thyroid glandular cells, including thyroglobulin proteolysis and iodide pumping, and it has a trophic influence on the thyroid, which results in an increase in the number and size of thyroid epithelial cells. Its secretion from the anterior pituitary is modulated by thyrotropin-releasing hormone, which is released from the hypothalamus, as well as by somatostatin, which has an inhibitory effect on TSH secretion. The effects of TSH on the thyroid are mediated by cyclic AMP, which is formed by adenyl cyclase following TSH receptor interaction. Most of the circulating thyroid hormone is bound to plasma proteins (albumin, globulin, and thyroxine-binding protein). TSH has no effect on the concentration of thyroxine-binding protein.

434. The answer is D. *(Ganong, 16/e, pp 391–393.)* Testosterone synthesis begins with the conversion of cholesterol to pregnenolone by stepwise hydroxylation. Pregnenolone is then converted to dehydroepiandrosterone, which can then undergo conversion to androstenedione and then to testosterone, a 17-hydroxysteroid. Estrogens can be formed from testosterone by stepwise reduction of the 3-keto group and ring aromatization. Those steps are irreversible; hence estrogen is not a precursor for testosterone.

435. The answer is C. *(Ganong, 16/e, pp 316–318.)* Glucagon is a peptide hormone secreted by the A (α) cells of the pancreatic islets. It acts to raise the blood glucose level. It also binds to receptors on liver cells and causes an increase in the cytosolic level of cyclic AMP. This stimulates the enzyme phosphorylase to break down glycogen into glucose. Glucagon does not stimulate glycogenolysis in muscle. It does stimulate the liver to make glucose from amino acids (gluconeogenesis) and increases lipolysis in adipose tissue. The fatty acids produced can then be taken up by the liver and be used to produce ketone bodies.

436. The answer is E. *(Ganong, 16/e, p 395. Guyton, 8/e, pp 896–897.)* Because gonadotropin secretion from the anterior pituitary gland is regulated by the secretion of gonadotropin-releasing hormone from the hypothalamus, it is not surprising that lesions in either of those sites would curtail gonadotropin production and result in hypogonadism. The pineal gland, located in the roof of the third ventricle, has been ascribed a variety of functions; it was originally described by Descartes as the seat of the soul. In animals, its activation by external light influences gonadotropin secretion. Although the function of the pineal gland in humans is unclear, pineal tumors are often associated with altered gonadotropin secretion. The testes are the major site of testosterone production. Testosterone is responsible for promoting and maintaining male secondary sex characteristics and sperm production.

437–443. The answers are 437-B, 438-A, 439-A, 440-C, 441-A, 442-B, 443-B. *(Berne, 3/e, pp 813–832.)* Hormones can be divided into two major groups on the basis of their mechanisms of action and biochemical properties: (1) the lipid-soluble hormones, which include adrenal (cortisol) and gonadal steroids, the iodothyronines (thyroxine), and vitamin D (cholecalciferol), and (2) the water-soluble peptide (LH, thyrotropin-releasing hormone, insulin) and catecholamine (epinephrine) hormones.

The lipid-soluble hormones, because of their limited water solubility, are transported in the plasma bound to proteins. They are able to penetrate the plasma membrane readily and interact with specific cytoplasmic receptors that solubilize them and transport them to the nucleus. Within the nucleus, the hormones act on specific receptors to stimulate the production of specific messenger RNA, which then directs the synthesis of specific protein products. These effects occur over a period of hours so that the physiologic response follows an initial lag period after hormone exposure. The mechanism by which these hormones influence nuclear function is still unclear. Characterization of cytoplasmic and nuclear receptors has indicated that they are proteins that bind their ligands with high specificity. The proteins have been partially purified and are characterized primarily by their ultracentrifugal sedimentation behavior and their affinity for their ligand.

The peptide and catecholamine hormones are water-soluble and circulate unbound in the plasma and extracellular fluid. These hormones bind to cell surface receptors in their target tissues and do not require penetration of the plasma membrane for their actions. In some cases, hormone-receptor complexes are internalized and degraded via lysosomal hydrolysis. Following interaction with their receptors, these hormones stimulate production of intracellular mediators, which function as "second messengers" for the "first messenger" (hormone). For many peptide and catecholamine hormones the intracellular messenger is a cyclic nucleotide, i.e., cyclic 3′,5′-adenosine monophosphate (cAMP) or cyclic 3′,5′-guanosine monophosphate (cGMP). The cyclic nucleotides are synthesized by membrane-bound nucleotide cyclases, which are coupled to hormone receptors by several intervening protein interactions. The cyclic nucleotides exert a variety of effects depending on the target tissue. The specificity of the hormone response is mediated by the hormone receptor and the metabolic capabilities of the target cell. Thus, although the two hormones luteinizing hormone and thyrotropin-releasing hormone both activate adenyl cyclase, they do so only in the target tissues that possess their receptors. One well-characterized mechanism of action of cyclic nucleotides is the activation of protein kinases to catalyze the phosphorylation of various protein substrates. Again, the specificity of the response depends on the properties of the target cell and the protein substrates available for phosphorylation. An example of this mechanism is the activation of phosphorylase in response to epinephrine in the liver.

A notable exception to the cyclic nucleotide second messenger mechanism is insulin, a polypeptide hormone that acts on a variety of target cells to alter carbohydrate, lipid, and protein metabolism. Although it is clear that insulin exerts its actions by binding to a plasma membrane receptor, the nature of its second messenger is still the subject of intense investigation.

It has been shown that another level of regulation characterizing hormone-sensitive systems involves the control of the number and affinity of receptors in the target cell membrane. Thus, changes in receptor number and density may be responsible for some of the diseases previously thought to result from an apparent deficiency in hormone secretion.

444–447. The answers are 444-B, 445-C, 446-D, 447-A. *(Ganong, 16/e, pp 221–222, 305–307, 385–387, 400–404.)* Breast development depends on the coordinated action of numerous hormones including prolactin, progesterone, estrogen, insulin, growth hormone, thyroid hormone, and glucocorticoids. The precise role of individual hormones is difficult to establish because each hormone may influence the secretion of others. In general, estrogens promote duct growth and progesterone and prolactin are essential for lobular development. The contributions of insulin, glucocorticoids, growth hormone, and thyroid hormone are not clear. Their presence appears to be necessary for breast development although some degree of breast function may occur in the presence of isolated deficiencies. Mineralocorticoids do not appear to be involved in breast development.

Oxytocin is a posterior pituitary peptide that promotes contraction of the myoepithelial cells surrounding breast ducts and causes expulsion of milk from lobular alveoli. Secretion of oxytocin is promoted by tactile stimulation of the breast by the nursing infant. It can also be elicited by psychic factors alone, such as the anticipation of nursing brought on by hearing the cry of the hungry infant. This anticipatory secretion of oxytocin may be experienced by the mother as a sensation of milk let-down in which milk appears at the nipple and may be forcibly ejected. Prolactin secretion is not subject to anticipatory psychic stimuli.

Estrogens, which play a complex role in mammary development, require the presence of growth hormone as well as prolactin. While promoting ductal development, estrogens actually inhibit lactation. The abrupt withdrawal of estrogen at parturition is one of the stimuli responsible for the onset of lactation. Nuclear and cytoplasmic estrogen receptors have been demonstrated in mammary tissue and have been used clinically to attempt to define the biologic potential for breast malignancy.

Progesterone receptors are also present in breast tissue. Progesterone acts synergistically with prolactin to promote lobular development.

448–450. The answers are 448-E, 449-A, 450-C. *(Berne, 3/e, pp 856–857, 859–862, 866–867. Ganong, 16/e, pp 305–313.)* Blood glucose levels are maintained by the actions of insulin and a variety of hormones that antagonize insulin action. Following oral intake of glucose, blood levels of glucose rise as glucose is absorbed from the gut (curve C in the graph accompanying the question). This rise in blood glucose level is not sustained because insulin secretion is stimulated. Insulin promotes glucose uptake into muscle and adipose tissue and thus reduces blood glucose concentration.

Administration of insulin without glucose results in hypoglycemia (curve E), a situation that occurs in diabetes mellitus when insulin injections are continued in the absence of adequate oral intake of glucose and that can lead to insulin shock. Severe depression of the brain—an organ that depends almost exclusively on glucose—may result from marked hypoglycemia and is a life-threatening situation that can be reversed by prompt infusion of glucose.

Alloxan is a β-cell antagonist that blocks glucose-stimulated insulin release and acts as a β-cell toxin. Thus, an alloxan-treated animal would manifest glucose tolerance similar to that of an insulin-deficient diabetic. Blood glucose would rise to very high levels because of limited glucose uptake in peripheral tissues in the absence of insulin (curve A).

451–455. The answers are 451-C, 452-E, 453-B, 454-A, 455-D. *(Ganong, 16/e, pp 302–303. West, 12/e, pp 754–755, 759.)* The endocrine pancreas consists of several hundred thousand nests of cells called islets of Langerhans. Most of these islets are located in the tail and body of the pancreas. The islets are entirely independent of the pancreatic ductal system and exocrine pancreas and secrete their hormones directly into the blood. The reason for the intimate physical relationship between endocrine and exocrine organs is unknown. In some lower species, they are anatomically separate.

The islets consist of at least four cell types, which can be distinguished by electron microscopy because their secretory granules are morphologically different. The cells can also be distinguished with the light microscope by immunohistochemical techniques. In these techniques, specific antibodies (e.g., rabbit anti-insulin) to the hormones are applied to microscopic sections of tissue (e.g., human pancreas), and their binding sites in the tissue are identified by applying a second antibody (e.g., goat antirabbit immunoglobulin) that is covalently linked to a fluorescent dye or enzyme that can be directly visualized following a nonspecific chemical reaction.

Morphological studies using these techniques have shown that the cells of the islets are not randomly distributed. The B (β) cells, which secrete insulin, are the most abundant and make up the central portion of the islets. These cells are recognized with the electron microscope by the β granules, which are membrane-bound organelles containing several rhomboid insulin crystals. The A (α) cells, which constitute about 20 percent of the cells, secrete glucagon. They form a layer around the central core of B (β) cells and are identified ultrastructurally by their α granules, which are membrane-bound organelles with an electron-dense core and peripheral electron-lucent halo. The D (δ) and F cells are also found near the rim of the islets and are in close proximity to both A (α) and B (β) cells. The D (δ) cells secrete somatostatin and the F cells secrete pancreatic polypeptide. Somatostatin released locally affects the secretion of both the A and B cells, an example of paracrine regulation. The precise physiologic role of pancreatic polypeptide, which is secreted in response to protein-containing meals and has plasma levels similar to those of glucagon, is still uncertain. In addition to paracrine mechanisms, local communication between islet cells may also occur through "gap" junctions, direct contact points of the cell membranes of the different cell types.

Secretin is secreted by cells in the duodenal mucosa and regulates pancreatic exocrine secretion. It is responsible primarily for bicarbonate and fluid secretion.

Neurophysiology

DIRECTIONS: Each question below contains five suggested responses. Select the **one best** response to each question.

456. The primary function of the bones of the middle ear in human hearing is to

(A) amplify the sound stimulus
(B) filter high-frequency sounds from the sound stimulus
(C) enable the direction of a sound stimulus to be detected
(D) enhance the ability to distinguish different sound frequencies
(E) protect the ear from damage

457. During a voluntary movement, the Golgi tendon organ provides the central nervous system with information about

(A) the length of the muscle being moved
(B) the velocity of the movement
(C) the blood flow to the muscle being moved
(D) the tension developed by the muscle being moved
(E) the change in joint angle produced by the movement

458. Repetitive stimulation of a skeletal muscle fiber will cause an increase in contractile strength because repetitive stimulation causes an increase in

(A) the duration of cross-bridge cycling
(B) the concentration of calcium in the myoplasm
(C) the magnitude of the end-plate potential
(D) the number of muscle myofibrils generating tension
(E) the velocity of muscle contraction

459. Which one of the following will most likely cause body temperature to remain about normal?

(A) A decrease in the amount of blood flowing to the skin
(B) An increase in the intensity of exercise
(C) An increase in the set point of the thermoregulatory system
(D) An increase in production of thyroxine
(E) A decrease in the amount of evaporative water loss

460. An aphasia is most likely to be associated with a lesion of

(A) the hippocampus
(B) Broca's area
(C) the parietal lobe
(D) the limbic system
(E) the reticular activating system

461. Which of the following structures is most responsible for the observation that not all frequencies of sound have the same threshold?

(A) Outer ear
(B) Middle ear
(C) Inner ear
(D) Tectorial membrane
(E) Basilar membrane

462. The most important role of the gamma motoneurons is to

(A) stimulate skeletal muscle fibers to contract
(B) maintain Ia afferent activity during contraction of muscle
(C) generate activity in Ib afferent fibers
(D) detect the length of resting skeletal muscle
(E) prevent muscles from producing too much force

463. The accompanying figure is a schematic diagram of a myoneural junction of a skeletal muscle. Substance 1 is the neurotransmitter released by the nerve that stimulates the muscle cell membrane to depolarize. With stimulation of the muscle cell membrane, ion 2 rushes intracellularly and ion 3 rushes extracellularly. Substances 1, 2, and 3 are, respectively,

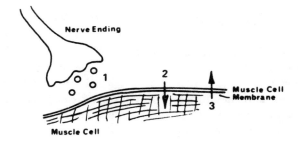

(A) acetylcholine, chloride, sodium
(B) acetylcholine, sodium, potassium
(C) acetylcholine, potassium, sodium
(D) norepinephrine, sodium, chloride
(E) norepinephrine, sodium, potassium

464. Which of the following determines whether release of neurotransmitter at synaptic junctions results in an excitatory or inhibitory effect on postsynaptic neurons?

(A) The chemical structure of the neurotransmitter
(B) The properties of the postsynaptic receptor
(C) The rate of reuptake of neurotransmitter by the presynaptic cell
(D) The amount of calcium released from presynaptic axons
(E) The velocity of axoplasmic transport in the presynaptic neuron

465. The middle cerebellar peduncle contains afferent fibers conveyed in which of the following tracts?

(A) Dorsal spinocerebellar
(B) Ventral spinocerebellar
(C) Tectocerebellar
(D) Pontocerebellar
(E) Vestibulocerebellar

466. The precentral gyrus and corticospinal tract are essential for

(A) vision
(B) olfaction
(C) auditory identification
(D) kinesthesia
(E) voluntary movement

467. A patient who presents with an intention tremor, scanning speech, "past-pointing," and a "drunken" gait might be expected to have a lesion involving the

(A) cerebellum
(B) medulla
(C) cortical motor strip
(D) basal ganglia
(E) eighth cranial nerve

468. Which of the following statements about the hair cells of the cochlea is true?

(A) They protect the lower airways from large particulate matter
(B) They support the basilar membrane
(C) They are connected by neural pathways to the lateral geniculate body
(D) They are contained in the macula
(E) They are vestigial organs without function

469. One of the reactions in the retinal rods directly caused by absorption of light energy is

(A) dissociation of scotopsin and metarhodopsin
(B) decomposition of scotopsin
(C) transformation of 11-*cis* retinal to all-*trans* retinal
(D) transformation of metarhodopsin to lumirhodopsin
(E) transformation of vitamin A to retinene

470. Which of the following statements about the cerebrospinal fluid (CSF) is true?

(A) It is absorbed by the choroid plexus
(B) Its absorption is independent of CSF pressure
(C) It circulates in the epidural space
(D) It has a lower glucose concentration than plasma
(E) It has a higher protein concentration than plasma

471. When a person slowly rotates toward the right,

(A) the stereocilia on the hair cells in the right horizontal semicircular canal bend away from the kinocilium
(B) both the left and right eyes deviate toward the left
(C) the hair cells in the left horizontal semicircular canal become depolarized
(D) the visual image on the retina becomes unfocused
(E) the endolymph in the left and right horizontal semicircular canals moves in opposite directions

472. Correct statements regarding rapid eye movement (REM) sleep include which of the following?

(A) It is the first state of sleep entered when a person falls asleep
(B) It is accompanied by loss of skeletal muscle tone
(C) It is characterized by a slow but steady heart rate
(D) It occurs more often in adults than in children
(E) It lasts longer than periods of slow-wave sleep

473. When emmetropic persons become presbyopic, their

(A) visual acuity increases
(B) near point increases
(C) far point decreases
(D) total refractive power increases
(E) ability to see distant objects decreases

474. When light strikes the eye, which of the following will increase?

(A) The sodium conductance of the photoreceptors
(B) The amount of transmitter released from the photoreceptors
(C) The concentration of rhodopsin in the photoreceptors
(D) The membrane potential of the photoreceptors
(E) The concentration of cyclic guanosine monophosphate (cGMP)

475. Spasticity can be caused by sectioning

(A) the corticospinal fibers
(B) the vestibulospinal fibers
(C) the Ia afferent fibers
(D) the corticoreticular fibers
(E) the reticulospinal fibers

476. Light shining on the retina will result in which of the following events?

(A) Activation of the nuclei of rod photoreceptors
(B) Conversion of guanosine triphosphate (GTP) to cyclic guanosine monophosphate (cGMP)
(C) Generation of *cis*-retinal from rhodopsin
(D) Depolarization of cone photoreceptors
(E) Activation of a phosphodiesterase enzyme

477. The cerebellum is important in controlling

(A) muscular coordination
(B) stereognosis
(C) muscle strength
(D) stretch reflexes
(E) posture

478. The alpha rhythm appearing on an electroencephalogram has which of the following characteristics?

(A) It produces 20 to 30 waves per second
(B) It disappears when a patient's eyes open
(C) It is replaced by slower, larger waves during REM sleep
(D) It represents activity that is most pronounced in the frontal region of the brain
(E) It is associated with deep sleep

479. Tapping the patella tendon elicits a reflex contraction of the quadriceps muscle. During the contraction of the quadriceps muscle,

(A) the Ib afferents from the Golgi tendon organ increase their rate of firing
(B) the Ia afferents from the muscle spindle increase their rate of firing
(C) the alpha motoneurons innervating the muscle spindles decrease their rate of firing
(D) the gamma motoneurons innervating the muscle spindles increase their rate of firing
(E) the alpha motoneurons to the antagonistic muscles increase their rate of firing

480. Visual accommodation involves which of the following mechanisms?

(A) Release of norepinephrine by sympathetic nerve fibers
(B) A decrease in the thickness of the lens
(C) Relaxation of the ciliary muscle
(D) Stretch of the lens suspensory ligaments
(E) A decrease in the focal length of the eye

481. Beta receptors activate G proteins that activate

(A) adenyl cyclase
(B) protein kinase A
(C) protein kinase C
(D) calmodulin
(E) phospholipase C

482. Norepinephrine will cause contraction of the smooth muscle in the

(A) bronchioles
(B) pupils
(C) intestine
(D) arterioles
(E) ciliary body

DIRECTIONS: Each numbered question or incomplete statement below is NEGATIVELY phrased. Select the **one best** lettered response.

483. All the following neurotransmitters are inactivated when diffused out of the cleft or pumped into the presynaptic nerve ending EXCEPT

(A) serotonin
(B) glycine
(C) norepinephrine
(D) dopamine
(E) acetylcholine

484. The hypothalamus is LEAST involved in the regulation of

(A) intake of water
(B) temperature
(C) osmolarity of urine
(D) respiration
(E) emotional behavior

485. Presynaptic inhibition in the central nervous system affects the sensitivity of motor neurons by inducing all the following changes EXCEPT

(A) an increase in the membrane conductance of the presynaptic nerve endings
(B) a decrease in the excitability of the α-motoneuron
(C) a partial depolarization of the presynaptic nerve endings
(D) a decrease in the firing rate of the α-motoneuron
(E) a decrease in the amount of mediator liberated at the synapse

486. The myotatic stretch reflex uses the smallest number of neurons of any cord reflex. Stretch of a muscle spindle causes all the following events EXCEPT

(A) excitation of receptors
(B) excitation of motor nerves
(C) transmission of impulses to anterior motor neurons
(D) a static as well as dynamic reflex
(E) relaxation of the muscle containing the muscle spindle

487. Mydriasis, or pupillary dilatation, involves all the following EXCEPT

(A) contraction of the radial fibers of the iris
(B) relaxation of the sphincter muscles of the iris
(C) stimulation of the Edinger-Westphal nucleus
(D) sympathetic nerve discharge
(E) impulse transmission by the superior cervical ganglion

488. All the following statements about the eye are true EXCEPT that the

(A) focal point of a hyperopic eye is behind the retina

(B) focal point of a myopic eye is in front of the retina

(C) focal point of an emmetropic eye is on the retina

(D) vision in a myopic eye can be corrected by use of a biconvex lens

(E) ciliary muscle is relaxed in an emmetropic eye focusing on an object 40 feet away

489. The vestibular apparatus is characterized by all the following EXCEPT

(A) the ability to detect linear acceleration via the macula

(B) the ability to detect angular acceleration via the cristae ampullaris

(C) the presence of endolymph in the membranous semicircular canals

(D) an afferent neural connection with the central nervous system via cranial nerve VIII

(E) the ability to produce a conscious sensation

DIRECTIONS: Each group of questions below consists of lettered headings followed by a set of numbered items. For each numbered item select the **one** lettered heading with which it is **most** closely associated. Each lettered heading may be used **once, more than once, or not at all.**

Questions 490–493

For each abnormality listed below, select the visual field defect (black area) that it is most likely to produce. Answer E if none of the options apply.

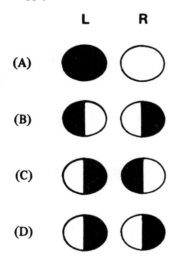

Questions 494–495

Match each description with one of the points on the action potential diagrammed below.

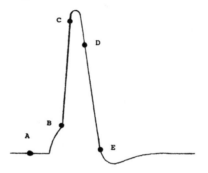

494. The point at which the driving force for potassium is the greatest

495. The point at which sodium conductance is greatest

490. Interruption of left optic nerve

491. Interruption of optic chiasma

492. Interruption of left optic tract

493. Enlargement of pituitary gland

Questions 496–500

Choose the brain region that is most closely associated with each of the pathophysiologic signs.

(A) Amygdala
(B) Flocculonodular lobe
(C) Occipital lobe
(D) Pons
(E) Posterior cerebellum

(F) Precentral gyrus
(G) Substantia nigra
(H) Subthalamic nucleus
(I) Temporal lobe
(J) Thalamus

496. Hemiballism

497. Rigidity

498. Intention tremor

499. Amnesia

500. Aphasia

Neurophysiology
Answers

456.   The answer is A. *(Berne, 3/e, pp 166–169.)* When sound waves pass from air to water, most of the energy contained in the sound stimulus is lost. Because the auditory receptors within the inner ear are bathed in liquid, most of the energy in the sound stimulus potentially could be lost as the sound travels from air to water. The bones of the middle ear significantly reduce the amount of loss by amplifying the sound stimulus. Most of the amplification results from the much larger surface area of the tympanic membrane compared with that of the oval window (or from the larger area of the malleus compared with that of the stapes). The reduction in area focuses the sound stimulus onto a smaller area, thus increasing the sound pressure. Audiologists refer to this amplification phenomenon as *impedance matching.*

457.   The answer is D. *(Berne, 3/e, pp 202–203. Ganong, 16/e, p 115.)* The Golgi tendon organ (GTO) is located in the tendon of skeletal muscles and therefore is in series with the muscle. Each time the muscle contracts, the tension developed by the muscle causes the GTO to be stretched. The Ib afferent fibers, which innervate the GTO, fire in proportion to the amount of GTO stretch, and therefore their firing rate provides the CNS with information about the amount of tension developed by the muscle. The muscle length and speed of shortening is sent to the CNS by Ia afferents that innervate the intrafusal fibers within muscle spindles.

458.   The answer is A. *(Berne, 3/e, pp 204–205.)* The maximal force that can be generated by a skeletal muscle fiber is determined by the number of cross bridges that are activated. Each time a skeletal muscle fiber is stimulated by an alpha motoneuron, enough Ca^{2+} is released from its sarcoplasmic reticulum (SR) to fully activate all the troponin within the muscle. Therefore, all the cross bridges can contribute to the generation of tension. However, the transmission of force from the cross bridges to the tendon (or bone or measuring device) does not occur until the series elastic component (SEC) of the muscle is stretched. Repetitive firing increases the amount of SEC stretch by maintaining cross-bridge cycling for a longer period of time. This occurs because each time the muscle is activated, the Ca^{2+} released from the SR replaces the CA^{2+} that has been resequestered since the last stimulus. Repetitive firing increases neither the concentration of Ca^{2+} within the myoplasm nor the number of myofibrils that are activated.

459. The answer is C. *(Berne, 3/e, pp 254–256. Guyton, 8/e, pp 797–805.)* When a person is exposed to a cold environment, the thermoregulatory system responds by activating a number of heat-conserving or heat-producing mechanisms. These include a decrease in blood supply to the skin, a decrease in sweating, an increase in shivering (or exercise), and an increase in metabolic activity brought about by an increase in shivering, exercise, or production of thyroxine. Although all of these mechanisms may increase body temperature above normal, they usually are evoked to bring body temperature back to normal. However, if the set point is increased (e.g., by a fever), the activity of the heat-conserving mechanisms will increase and those mechanisms that bring about a loss of heat will decrease, which will cause a rise in temperature.

460. The answer is B. *(Berne, 3/e, p 271. Guyton 8/e, pp 640–642.)* Aphasia is a language disorder in which a person is unable to properly express or understand certain aspects of written or spoken language. It is caused by lesions to the language centers of the brain, which, for the majority of persons, are located within the left hemisphere in the portions of the temporal and frontal lobes known as Wernicke's and Broca's areas, respectively. Language disorders caused by memory loss, which could be the result of a hippocampal lesion, are not classified as aphasias.

461. The answer is B. *(Berne, 3/e, pp 166–173.)* In order for sounds to be detected by the ear, they must pass from the air to the fluid medium of the inner ear. For this to occur, the sound pressure must be amplified (or an impedance match between air and fluid must be created). The large difference in surface area between the tympanic membrane and oval window of the middle ear provides for this amplification (or impedance matching). However, not all frequencies are equally amplified; certain frequencies, those between 500 and 5000 Hz, are heard at much lower sound pressures than are lower or higher frequencies.

462. The answer is B. *(Berne, 3/e, pp 198–202.)* The gamma motoneurons innervate the intrafusal fibers of the muscle spindles. When a skeletal muscle contracts, the intrafusal muscle fiber becomes slack and the Ia afferents stop firing. By stimulating the intrafusal muscle fibers during a contraction, the gamma motoneurons prevent the intrafusal muscle fibers from becoming slack and thus maintain Ia firing during the contraction.

463. The answer is B. *(Berne, 3/e, pp 55–59.)* At rest, the difference in electrical potential across the membrane of the muscle cell (resting potential) is −90 millivolts. The nerve releases acetylcholine, which changes the ionic permeability of the muscle plasma membrane. Owing to the differences in concentration of sodium ions (high outside) and potassium ions (high inside) across the membrane, the increased permeability to ions gives rise to a sudden influx of sodium and efflux of potassium ions through the plasma membrane. This results in depolarization of the muscle membrane.

464. The answer is B. *(Berne, 3/e, pp 61–68.)* Release of neurotransmitter from presynaptic cells is accompanied by an influx of calcium from the extracellular fluid. The neurotransmitter then interacts with receptors on the plasma membrane of the postsynaptic cell. It is the specificity of these receptors that determines whether the net effect is inhibitory or excitatory. A specific transmitter may have either effect depending on the site of action. Thus, acetylcholine is excitatory at the neuromuscular junction but is inhibitory when released by the vagus nerve at cardiac muscle junctions.

465. The answer is D. *(Berne, 3/e, pp 229–239.)* The middle cerebellar peduncle contains afferent fibers conveyed in the pontocerebellar tract, which carries impulses from the motor area as well as other parts of the cerebellar cortex except the flocculonodular lobe. The dorsal spinocerebellar and vestibulocerebellar afferent tracts enter the cerebellum via the inferior peduncle. The ventral spinocerebellar and tectocerebellar tracts enter via the superior cerebellar peduncle.

466. The answer is E. *(Berne, 3/e, pp 212–219.)* The precentral gyrus is the motor area of the cortex and the corticospinal tract is the pyramidal tract proper. These two structures are essential for voluntary movement. A supplementary motor area, whose function is still unknown, exists on the medial side of the hemisphere.

467. The answer is A. *(Berne, 3/e, pp 229–243.)* Ataxia, scanning speech, dysmetria, and an intention tremor all are classic findings in a patient with a lesion involving the cerebellum. Affected persons also exhibit adiadochokinesia, which is a loss of ability to accomplish a swift succession of oscillatory movements, such as external and internal rotation of the foot. These symptoms all result from destruction of the normal feedback mechanisms that are coordinated in the cerebellum.

468. The answer is D. *(Berne, 3/e, pp 169–175.)* The cochlear hair cells are the functioning auditory receptors. Neural pathways from the hair cells pass to the inferior colliculi and the medial geniculate body before synapsing in the auditory cortex. The hair cells are contained in the macula (otolithic organ) and are overlaid by the otolithic membrane.

469. The answer is C. (*Berne, 3/e, pp 147–152. Guyton, 8/e, pp 548–550.*) The light-sensitive chemical in the retinal rods is called *rhodopsin*. It is a combination of retinal (in the 11-*cis* configuration) and opsin. Light immediately changes the 11-*cis* structure of retinal to the all-*trans* structure. Other reactions follow because the physical structure of the all-*trans* retinal no longer combines in a stable fashion with opsin. Rhodopsin's decomposition upon exposure to light excites the nerve fibers in the eye.

470. The answer is D. (*Berne, 3/e, pp 96–97. Guyton, 8/e, pp 681–684.*) Cerebrospinal fluid (CSF), which is in osmotic equilibrium with the extracellular fluid of the brain and spinal cord, is formed primarily in the choroid plexus by an active secretory process. It circulates through the subarachnoid space between the dura mater and pia mater and is absorbed into the circulation by the arachnoid villi. The epidural space, which lies outside the dura mater, may be used clinically for instillation of anesthetics. CSF protein and glucose concentrations are much lower than those of plasma. Changes in those concentrations in the CSF are helpful in detecting pathologic processes, e.g., tumor or infection, in which the blood-brain barrier is disrupted.

471. The answer is B. (*Berne, 3/e, pp 179–186. Guyton, 8/e, pp 681–684.*) When the head rotates in one direction, the hair cells mounted on the cristae rotate along with the head. However, the flow of endolymph is delayed and as a result the cupula is moved in a direction opposite to the movement of the head. When the head moves to the right, the cupula moves toward the left; this bends the stereocilia on the hair cells in the right horizontal canal toward the kinocilium and bends the stereocilia on the hair cells in the left horizontal canal toward the kinocilium. As a result the hair cells in the right horizontal canal depolarize and those in the left horizontal canal hyperpolarize. The depolarization of the hair cells in the right horizontal canal stimulates the right vestibular nerve, which in turn causes the eyes to deviate toward the left. The movement of the eyes toward the left as the head deviates toward the right keeps the image on the retina in focus.

472. The answer is B. (*Berne, 3/e, pp 269–270.*) In a normal sleep cycle, a person passes through the four stages of slow-wave sleep before entering REM sleep. In narcolepsy, a person may pass directly from the waking state to REM sleep. REM sleep is characterized by irregular heart beats and respiration and by periods of atonia (loss of muscle tone). It is also the state of sleep in which dreaming occurs.

473. The answer is B. (*Berne, 3/e, pp 145–146. Guyton, 8/e, pp 538–539.*) In presbyopia, the ability of the lens to accommodate for near vision decreases.

Thus the total refractive power of the eye decreases and the ability of the eye to form a focused image of objects placed close to it decreases. The near point is the closest point to which an object can be brought and still remain in focus. This increases when the accommodative power of the eye is decreased. There is no effect on the far point or visual acuity; these remain normal.

474.   The answer is D. *(Berne, 3/e, pp 147–152. Guyton, 8/e, pp 548–550.)* When light strikes the eye and is absorbed by rhodopsin, a photoisomerization of 11-*cis* retinal to all-*trans* retinal occurs. As a consequence of this photoisomerization, rhodopsin is activated. The rhodopsin then activates transducin, which in turn activates a phosphodiesterase, which hydrolyzes cGMP. When cGMP concentrations within the rods or cones decrease, sodium channels close, sodium conductance decreases, and the cell hyperpolarizes. Hyperpolarization of the cell causes a decrease in the release of neurotransmitter. Eventually the all-*trans* retinal dissociates from opsin and reduces the concentration of rhodopsin n the cell.

475.   The answer is D. *(Ganong, 16/e, pp 115–117, 184, 186–188, 190–191.)* Spasticity results from overactivity of the alpha motoneurons innervating the skeletal musculature. Under normal circumstances, these alpha motoneurons are tonically stimulated by reticulospinal and vestibulospinal fibers originating in the brainstem. These brainstem fibers are normally inhibited by fibers originating in the cortex. Cutting the cortical fibers releases the brainstem fibers from inhibition and results in spasticity. Cutting the fibers from the reticular formation or vestibular nuclei or the Ia afferents will reduce the spasticity.

476.   The answer is E. *(Berne, 3/e, pp 147–152. Guyton, 8/e, pp 548–550.)* The retina contains two types of photoreceptors: rods, which function in gray level discrimination, and cones, which are important in light and color vision. These receptor cells derive their names from their shapes, and their shapes are determined by their complex plasma membrane, which comprises hundreds to thousands of disk-shaped structures containing photopigments. When light shines on the retina, it interacts with these disks and causes *cis-trans* isomerization of retinal, the prosthetic group associated with the photoreceptor proteins. This isomerization is associated with hydrolysis of cGMP by a light-sensitive cGMP phosphodiesterase and with hyperpolarization of the plasma membrane caused by a decrease in sodium conductance across the membrane. The nucleus of the photoreceptor cell has no known role in the response to light.

477.   The answer is A. *(Berne, 3/e, pp 229–237.)* The primary function of the cerebellum is to coordinate muscular activity throughout the body. It does so without directly controlling muscular contraction but by receiving input from the periphery and cerebral motor areas and comparing the actual position of each part of the body with the position intended by motor centers. Pain sensation is mediated by afferent fibers that interact primarily with the thalamus and parietal cortex. Stereognosis, the recognition of objects by touch without vision, is mediated by the cortex.

478. The answer is B. *(Berne, 3/e, pp 268–270.)* In a totally relaxed adult with eyes closed, the major component of the electroencephalogram (EEG) will be a regular pattern of 8 to 12 waves per second, called the *alpha rhythm.* The alpha rhythm disappears when the eyes are opened. It is most prominent in the parietooccipital region. In deep sleep, the alpha rhythm is replaced by larger, slower waves called *delta waves.* In REM sleep, the EEG will show fast, irregular activity.

479. The answer is A. *(Berne, 3/e, pp 198–205.)* Stretching the patella tendon stretches the muscle spindles within the quadriceps muscle and causes an increase in Ia afferent activity. The increase in Ia afferent activity causes an increase in alpha motoneuron activity, which results in contraction of the quadriceps muscle. When the muscle contracts, the muscle spindles are unloaded and the Ia afferent activity is reduced. However, the Ib activity is increased during contraction because of the tension placed on the Golgi tendon organs.

480. The answer is E. *(Berne, 3/e, pp 144–146. Guyton, 8/e, pp 534–541.)* When an object is brought nearer to the eye, it is kept in focus by increasing the refractive power of the eye. Increasing the refractive power of the eye causes a decrease in the focal length. Refractive power is increased by the accommodation reflex, which is initiated by parasympathetic fibers that contract the ciliary muscle. This allows the suspensory ligaments to retract, which in turn permits the lens to thicken and increase its curvature. The increase in curvature causes the increase in the refractive power of the eye.

481. The answer is A. *(Berne, 3/e, pp 80–85.)* Beta-receptor activated G proteins activate adenyl cyclase, which catalyzes the production of cAMP from ATP. The cAMP then activates protein kinase A, which produces its physiologic effects by phosphorylating a variety of proteins. Phospholipase C is activated by a G protein, which is activated by muscarinic and alpha$_1$-adrenergic receptors. Phospholipase C hydrolyzes PIP$_2$ and thus produces IP$_3$ and DAG. Protein kinase C is in turn activated by DAG.

482. The answer is D. *(Berne, 3/e, pp 80–85, 244–246, 250.)* The catecholamines norepinephrine and epinephrine will activate both alpha- and beta-adrenergic receptors. When the alpha$_1$-adrenergic receptors are stimulated they activate a G protein, which in turn activates phospholipase C that hydrolyzes PIP$_2$ and produces IP$_3$ and DAG. The IP$_3$ causes the release of Ca^{2+} from the sarcoplasmic reticulum, which in turn increases muscle contraction. Alpha$_1$-adrenergic receptors predominate on arteriolar smooth muscle, so these muscles contract when stimulated with norepinephrine. The bronchiolar, pupillary, and ciliary smooth muscles all contain beta receptors, which cause smooth muscle relaxation. The intestinal smooth muscle relaxation is initiated by an alpha$_2$-adrenergic receptor.

483. The answer is E. *(Ganong, 16/e, pp 87–95.)* The action of acetylcholine (ACh) is terminated by acetylcholinesterase (AChE), which hydrolyzes ACh to acetate and choline. The choline is pumped into the nerve terminal and used in the resynthesis of new ACh. All other transmitters are inactivated by reuptake into the nerve terminal. A variety of drugs act by preventing reuptake of the neurotransmitter into the nerve terminal or, in the case of ACh, by blocking the action of AChE.

484. The answer is D. *(Berne, 3/e, pp 254–257.)* The hypothalamus contains osmoreceptors responsible for detecting increases in extracellular osmolarity. These osmoreceptors produce the sensation of thirst, increase drinking, and cause the release of antidiuretic hormone (ADH). Thermoreceptors in the anterior hypothalamus measure core temperature. Other hypothalamic neurons are involved in the initiation and coordination of heat-conserving and heat-losing mechanisms. The hypothalamus also serves as a component of the limbic system, which is responsible, in part, for mediating emotional behavior. Respiration is controlled by respiratory centers of the brainstem.

485. The answer is A. *(Berne, 3/e, p 68.)* Presynaptic inhibition is caused by interneurons that secrete a transmitter that increases Cl$^-$conductance of the presynaptic nerve ending. This increase in membrane conductance causes a partial depolarization of the presynaptic nerve ending and a decrease in the magnitude of the action potential in the presynaptic nerve ending. Because the amount of mediator released at the synapse is related to the magnitude of the action potential, less transmitter is released and the firing rate of the postsynaptic α-motoneuron is decreased. Presynaptic inhibition does not change the membrane potential of the α-motoneuron, and therefore the excitability of the α-motoneuron is not affected.

486. The answer is E. *(Berne, 3/e, pp 203–205.)* The myotatic (stretch) reflex, which is a spinal cord reflex that prevents further stretch of muscle by stimulating contraction of muscle fiber, is important in preventing oscillation and jerking movements. It is mediated by a specialized muscle fiber, the muscle spindle, which, when stretched, transmits impulses via the dorsal root to motor neurons in the anterior horn of the spinal cord. The reflex is normally subject to both facilitation and inhibition by higher centers.

487. The answer is C. (*West, 12/e, pp 972, 975–976.*) Sympathetic nerves from the superior cervical ganglion innervate the radial fibers of the iris, and their excitation induces pupillary dilatation. Constriction of the pupil in response to light is mediated via afferent fibers to the pretectal area of the pons, from which efferent fibers pass to the nucleus of Edinger-Westphal. From that point, parasympathetic cholinergic fibers pass via the ciliary ganglion to the ciliary muscles and sphincter of the iris. When dilatation of the pupil occurs, the nucleus of Edinger-Westphal is inhibited.

488. The answer is D. (*Berne, 3/e, pp 143–146. Guyton, 8/e, pp 534–541.*) Biconcave (not biconvex) lenses cause light rays to diverge and, when placed in front of a myopic (nearsighted) eye, will move the focal point back until it reaches the retina, which is required to correct nearsightedness. In hyperopia (farsightedness), the eyeball is decreased in anteroposterior diameter, resulting in a focal point that lies *behind* the retina; in myopia, this diameter is increased, causing the focal point to lie in *front* of the retina. Emmetropia refers to an optically normal eye. In astigmatism, another common refractive error, the curvature of the cornea is nonspherical.

489. The answer is E. (*Berne, 3/e, pp 179–186.*) In the vestibular apparatus the macula is located in the utricle and the cristae ampullaris are located in the ampullae of the semicircular canals. The macula and the cristae ampullaris have similar structures containing hair cells that are stimulated by otoconia. Maculae, being sensitive to changes in gravitational pull, are able to detect *linear* acceleration; ampullar structures, being sensitive to changes in the flow of endolymph in the semicircular canals, are able to detect *angular* acceleration. Sensory nerve fibers are transmitted via cranial nerve VIII to the vestibular nuclei. Although the vestibular apparatus produces a feeling of up and down and of movement, no particular conscious sensation results from vestibular nerve activity.

490–493. The answers are 490-A, 491-B, 492-D, 493-B. (*Berne, 3/e, pp 156–160.*) The visual pathway consists of the retina, optic nerve, optic chiasma, optic tract, and visual (or occipital) cerebral cortex, in that order. The spatial relationships of fibers in the retina are maintained in the pattern of fibers leaving the eye via the optic nerve: fibers representing the temporal retina (nasal field) stay on the same side and fibers representing the nasal retina (temporal field) cross at the optic chiasma.

Defects in the field of vision can result from primary diseases of the retina or interruption of the optic pathway. Defects caused by primary retinal disease or vascular disease (hypertension or diabetes) often begin at the periphery of vision and may produce numerous small defects, or scotomata. Visual field analysis can be employed to localize lesions in the optic pathway that are causing blindness. Thus, a lesion involving the optic chiasma will block impulses from the nasal halves of both retinae to produce bitemporal hemianopia (choice B in the question). Such lesions are most commonly caused by pituitary tumors. The pituitary gland is situated in the sella turcica immediately beneath the optic chiasma, from which it is separated by a dural membrane, the diaphragma sellae. Enlargement of the pituitary by tumor or infiltrative processes frequently results in upward expansion, causing compression of the optic chiasma and interruption of the decussating fibers from the nasal retinae.

Interruption of one optic nerve will clearly produce total blindness in the affected eye (choice A). Besides trauma, other processes that may cause optic nerve deficits include orbital tumors or compromise of the blood supply.

Interruption of an optic tract beyond the optic chiasma would denervate the half of the retina on the same side as the lesion and produce a contralateral visual defect referred to a homonymous hemianopia (choice D). The defect illustrated in choice C, in which there is loss of nasal fields bilaterally, could not occur from a lesion at a single site.

494–495. The answers are 494-C, 495-C. *(Berne, 3/e, pp 33–34, 38–40.)* The driving force for an ion is the sum of the electrical and diffusional forces acting on the ion. The driving force is calculated from the formula $E_M - E_{ion}$, where E_M is the membrane potential and E_{ion} is the Nernst, or equilibrium, potential for the ion. Based on this formula, the driving force for an ion is greatest when the difference between the membrane potential and the equilibrium potential for that ion is greatest. Since E_K (equilibrium potential for potassium) is −92 mV, the driving force is greatest when the membrane is most positive. In this case, this is at point C. The upstroke of the action potential is caused by an increase in sodium conductance. Sodium conductance begins to increase at threshold (point B) and reaches a maximum near the peak of the action potential (point C). Points B through D are part of the absolute refractory period. During this period, a second action potential cannot occur. Point E is part of the relative refractory period. During this period a second action potential can be generated, but the stimulus strength must be greater than normal. When the net ionic fluxes across a membrane are zero, the membrane potential is not changing. Such a situation occurs when the cell is at the resting potential (point A) and at the peaks of the overshoot and undershoot.

496–500. The answers are 496-H, 497-G, 498-E, 499-I, 500-I. *(Berne, 3/e, pp 238–242. Ganong, 16/e, pp 193–200.)* Hemiballism is characterized by wild flinging movements of the extremities. It is produced by lesions within the subthalamus and its signs are expressed on the side opposite to the lesion.

Rigidity is one of the classic signs of Parkinson's disease. The rigidity is described as cogwheel rigidity because the resistance to movement disappears while the limb is being passively moved and reappears when the limb becomes still. In this regard, it differs from the spasticity associated with upper motor neuron disease. In spasticity, the resistance to movement steadily increases as the limb is being passively moved. In addition to rigidity, patients suffering from Parkinson's disease also display resting tremors, which disappear during movements, and bradykinesia (the inability to make rapid movements). Parkinsonism is characterized by a loss of melanin-containing nerve cells from the substantia nigra.

In contrast to patients who have Parkinson's disease and who display spontaneous resting tremors, those who have had lesions within their posterior cerebellum produce tremors only while they are carrying out a goal-directed movement. These tremors are called *intention tremors* because they occur when the limb is intentionally being moved.

The hippocampus is part of the limbic lobe, which is formed from the medial parts of the temporal, parietal, and frontal lobes. The hippocampus is intimately associated with memory, and lesions within this area of the brain will lead to a variety of memory disorders including amnesia.

Aphasia is defined as the inability to understand (receptive, or Wernicke's, aphasia) or generate (expressive, or Broca's, aphasia) the motor pattern necessary for speech. Receptive aphasia is caused by lesions within the temporal lobe that affect Wernicke's speech area. It is a cognitive rather than a motor control disorder; that is, there are no deficits in the ability of the person to utilize the muscles involved in normal speech. Interestingly, patients who communicate by signing rather than hearing lose their ability to communicate when the speech areas in their left hemisphere are damaged.

Bibliography

Johnson LR (ed): Essentials of Medical Physiology. New York, Raven, 1992.

Berne RM, Levy MN: *Physiology*, 2/e. St. Louis, CV Mosby, 1988.

Ganong WF: *Review of Medical Physiology*, 16/e. East Norwalk, CT, Appleton & Lange, 1994.

Guyton, AC: *Textbook of Medical Physiology*, 8/e. Philadelphia, WB Saunders, 1991.

Rose BD: *Clinical Physiology of Acid-Base and Electrolyte Disorders*, 4/e. New York, McGraw-Hill, 1994.

West JB: *Best and Taylor's Physiological Basis of Medical Practice*, 12/e. Baltimore, Williams & Wilkins, 1990.

West JB: *Respiratory Physiology: The Essentials*, 5/e. Baltimore, Williams & Wilkens, 1995.